EAT
YOURSELF
BEAUTIFUL

GW00357176

Liz Earle EAT YOURSELF BEAUTIFUL

BBC BOOKS

This book has been published to accompany the
BBC television series entitled *Eat Yourself Beautiful*

Published by BBC Books,
a division of BBC Enterprises Limited
Woodlands, 80 Wood Lane
London W12 0TT

First published 1992

ISBN 0 563 36392 4

Set in Century Old Style by
Phoenix Photosetting, Chatham, Kent
Printed and bound in Great Britain by
Clays Ltd, St Ives plc
Cover printed by Clays Ltd, St Ives plc

For Lily

Beauty lies in the health of her generation

About the author

Liz Earle is a popular television presenter and best-selling author with a special interest in health and beauty. She has presented her own highly successful series, *Beautywise*, on BBC 1 and is a regular contributor to television and radio. The former health and beauty editor of *New Woman* magazine, Liz has a wealth of specialist knowledge and a compelling enthusiasm for promoting better health. She shares with medics and nutritionists a firm belief in the fundamental value of nutrition. Her previous books include *Vital Oils* and *Save Your Skin with Vital Oils* (Vermilion). Liz Earle lives in London and Gloucestershire with her husband Patrick and daughter Lily.

CONTENTS

Acknowledgements

While writing this book I have been fortunate to work with many health professionals whom I admire and respect. I should like to thank all those who gave their time so generously and who shared their valuable knowledge with me. In particular, I should like to thank Michael Skipwith for his naturopathic guidance and recipes. Also Eleanor Hale for ideas that prove wholefood really does taste delicious! A special thank you to my agent Rosemary Sandberg and to my researcher Annie Bawtree. My gratitude also to Suzanne Webber and Cyril Gates at the BBC for their confidence and encouragement. There is no doubt that we can all eat ourselves healthy as well as beautiful. From research professors to politicians, there are many involved in the issues that need to be tackled to encourage better health and well-being. Our health and beauty are our future – they are too important to ignore.

INTRODUCTION

Beauty is about better health. It is about clear, radiant skin and a sparkle in the eye. Without better health there can be no beauty. Good health encourages the energy and vitality that give us our glowing good looks. This book is about improving the way we look and feel by simply watching what we eat. Our diet provides the fuel for every living cell in the body, and knowing what foods to eat makes a dramatic difference to our appearance. The *only* way to improve significantly the way we look is from within – literally to feed our face.

The simple guidelines I've described in this book can bring about staggering beauty benefits. After just six weeks you can expect:

A brighter, clearer complexion
Smoother, stronger skin
Greater resistance to the signs of ageing
Fewer spots and skin disorders
Shiny, more manageable hair
Longer, stronger nails

Outward beauty is fundamentally linked to good health and the only way to boost this is from the inside. Eating yourself beautiful not only enhances your appearance but also encourages the very best of health. These are just a few of the many differences you will see:

Increased energy and zest for life

Less sign of stress

A stronger immune system

Fewer inflammatory disorders such as arthritis

Relief from PMT and menopausal problems

Greater resistance to heart disease

This eating plan was tested by a group of volunteers over a six-week period. These are just a few of their genuine comments:

'I had far fewer skin problems. My skin began to look healthier and I noticed a reduction in cellulite.'

'There was a definite improvement in my energy levels and my general health. I lost a stone in weight, felt much more energetic, slept more soundly and was able to get up more quickly in the morning!'

'I felt much better, my skin improved, others thought I looked healthier.'

'I slept better, my skin was less greasy, I had improved energy levels and lost half a stone.'

'I noticed changes in my skin, people said I looked brighter and healthier. I had lots of energy and lost about 4 lb.'

> *'I had more energy and lost half a stone.'*
>
> *'My skin was clearer and my weight decreased.'*
>
> *'A colleague said I looked "much younger". I thought my skin looked better, I felt extremely energetic and I lost some weight.'*

This book is the key to unlocking your inner beauty. The ideas are straightforward, inexpensive and best of all – it works! You may never know the benefits unless you give it a try.

Liz Earle

EAT YOURSELF BEAUTIFUL

Eating the right kind of food has an enormous impact on the way our body looks and behaves. The link between diet, good looks and better health has been established for many years. Worldwide medical research now confirms what health practitioners have known for thousands of years – *you are what you eat*. This book reveals several important studies into specific foods and the results may surprise you. From a softer complexion to stronger nails and shinier hair, all metabolic processes depend on diet. Skin cells in particular rely on a balanced supply of nutrients to grow, strengthen and fight the degenerative ageing processes. Far more effective than any skin cream, the real power to turn back the clock comes from within.

The fact that natural substances have the power to rejuvenate, repair and re-shape the body is nothing new. Many ancient remedies are backed by modern science and some hi-tech medicines have their roots firmly in the past. For example, aspirin comes from the willow tree, while *digitalis* is one of our most powerful drugs for heart disease and is extracted from the common foxglove. The therapeutic properties of foods are also being documented as scientists discover that many foods have powerful healing properties. The most important groups of foods are the wholegrains, fruits, vegetables, oils and herbs. Each is explored in more detail in future chapters with notes at the back of the book for some of the longer medical references. Meanwhile, here is a taste of just a few of the benefits in store:

Oatbran and the pectin in many fruits consist of soluble fibre which is known to control cholesterol. The insoluble fibre found in wholegrains and many vegetables holds water within the colon, carries waste matter out of the body and prevents constipation.

Nuts and seeds are highly concentrated sources of energy and also house a few surprises. A one-month trial reported in the American Journal of Clinical Nutrition *shows that adding 2 oz (50 g) of almonds to a low-fat diet can reduce cholesterol levels by an average of 11 per cent* further *than a low-fat diet alone.*

Cranberries are nature's cure for bladder and urinary tract infections (more about their properties on page 96). According to Professor Sobota, a microbiologist at Youngstown State University in Ohio, they are also a powerful natural antibiotic.

Cabbage juice has been used in America, Germany and India to treat peptic stomach ulcers successfully.

Fish oils extracted from herrings, mackerel and salmon are prescribed by cardiologists worldwide to treat heart disease. The nutrients found in these fatty fish have also been shown to improve serious skin disorders, including psoriasis.

Olive oil lowers your risk of heart disease and can improve the texture of your skin. Evening primrose oil has also been clinically proven to improve dry skin conditions such as eczema and a version is available on prescription.

> *Garlic fights bacteria within the skin and kills fungal infections. Its powerful anti-bacterial properties also protect us from coughs and colds and it is proven that it helps prevent blood clots and high cholesterol levels.*

Some foods have a more direct impact on our appearance: substances found in unrefined avocado oil have been shown to increase the production of soluble collagen within the skin (1). This type of skin protein makes up the fibres that support the skin and is essential to keep our faces smooth and elastic. Insufficient supplies are the major reason why our skin slackens and sags with age. So the key to a clear complexion could be found in a simple salad instead of a jar of skin cream. Avocados are not the only foods to have an anti-ageing action. Many other foods contain the vital vitamins, minerals and trace elements that also have specific skin-enhancing actions. Vitamin C, vitamin E, vitamin B6 and calcium are all required for healthy collagen metabolism within the skin.

Other nutrients needed to keep the complexion smooth are the essential fatty acids (EFAs). These include linoleic acid which makes up around 70 per cent of the skin. If the body falls short of EFAs, our skin quickly becomes dry and fine lines and wrinkles become more visible. This is why even those following a strictly low-fat diet need to include a small amount of natural oils in their foods every day. Essential fatty acids can be found in nuts, seeds and vegetables as well as the richer plant and fish oils. These substances have been used for many years to treat skin disorders and there are over 200 studies recorded on the effect of EFAs on skin conditions as diverse as acne and eczema. More about the remarkable healing powers of natural oils in chapter five. Meanwhile, it is clear that many nutrients have a profound effect on our appearance and it really is possible to eat yourself beautiful.

How To Eat Yourself Beautiful

The idea of eating yourself beautiful is nothing new and can be traced back to the earliest civilisations. Renowned physicians of every era have recognised the fundamental effect food has on our looks and wellbeing. The ancient dynasties of East Asia believed that human health depended on diet alone and even the great Chinese sage Confucius contended that food is a major cause of disorders in the body and advised against eating too much meat and rich, processed foods. Buddha also believed that good health could only be achieved by diet and cautioned against eating meat while advocating grains as a purifying, life-enhancing food.

Variety is the spice of life and there is evidence that eating a varied diet is the best way to build the body beautiful. The ancient Chinese five-taste theory of inner energy claims that the five flavours of sweet, sour, bitter, salty and spicy correspond to different organs and areas in the body. Eating too much food from one family overloads and eventually weakens its corresponding organ or function. Unfortunately, our Western diet now relies far too heavily on the high fat, high sugar, refined foods. The secret to eating yourself beautiful is simple. We need a varied, balanced diet of fresh, whole foods and our daily diet should include generous portions of grains, fresh fruit and vegetables, unrefined oils, herbs and spices. This is why it is the *quality* of food that is eaten, and not the *quantity*, that is so important. You should eat sufficient quantities of food to feel comfortably full and not agonise unduly over portion sizes. But before we begin to enjoy the right kinds of foods we must first give our body a break from all our bad habits.

And Now . . .
The Eat Yourself Beautiful Guidelines!

The guidelines for eating well are simple: fresh, whole foods pre-pared with the minimum of processing. As the basis of your diet try to include these foods.

Eat daily:

Wholegrains	*2 or more types*
Fresh fruit	*2 or more varieties*
Vegetables	*3 or more varieties (in addition to potatoes)*
Unrefined oils	*1 tablespoonful*
Herbs and spices	*2 or more types*

The reason why potatoes do not count as a vegetable is that they are nutritionally classified as a starchy food, so you need to eat three kinds of vegetables other than potatoes. The regime is not strictly vegetarian and you may add small amounts of meat, fish and eggs. But watch out for cooked meat products such as pies, sausages, burgers and tinned meat. Most are likely to contain mechanically recovered meat (MRM) which is legally allowed to include head meat such as ears, eyelids and brain, offal including heart and lungs, stomach, tail meat, tongue and testicles. Yum yum. And if you think of meat as the lean part of an animal with all the fat and gristle trimmed away, think again. The laws covering the making of sausages permit fat and connective tissue (skin, rind, sinew and gristle) to be declared legally as part of the 'meat' content. Up to 50 per cent of your average banger may be made of connective tissue and fat. Other undesirable extras include phosphates added to hold water in the sausage, colours to improve its 'meaty' appearance, and preservatives to stop the fat from turning rancid and to increase shelf life. A 1990 survey carried out by The Consumer's Association found all but one brand of sausages (made by the Real Meat company) contained sulphites (E220 to E227) which are known to cause allergic reactions. No wonder nine million Britons are avoiding red meat.

Milk and dairy produce tend to be high in saturated fat and are also highly mucus-forming so they should be limited. Many people are either intolerant of wheat or too wheat-dependent, so for the first few weeks it is a good idea to restrict your intake of wheat-based products such as bread and pasta or even cut them out altogether. Processed and packaged foods may be included to a limited extent but make sure you read **every** label and know **exactly** what you're eating. Be aware that some labelling can mislead simply by the information that is left out. If a packet boldly states, 'no artificial colour or flavouring', you can be sure it contains a chemical preservative. A packet that emphasises 'low-fat' on the front may bury its high sugar content in small print on the back. Sometimes chemical names are used instead of E numbers as manufacturers have realised that the consumer is rightly wary of these.

Because these guidelines reduce many of the common allergens such as wheat, dairy products and additives, those who suffer from allergy-related symptoms (whether they recognise them or not) will automatically find their wellbeing improves. There is so much to be gained – so what are you waiting for? Take control of your looks and well-being simply by watching what you eat.

The Vital Vitamins

THE ANTI-AGER

Vitamin A is sometimes called the 'skin vitamin' as it is needed to repair skin tissues, and low levels in our diet lead to spots, acne and a scaly scalp. Vitamin A is also essential for good eyesight and improves the immune system. Of the many studies into vitamin A, one recorded in the *Australian Paediatric Journal* shows that children given daily supplements of vitamin A (equivalent to the amount in half a carrot) had far fewer respiratory illnesses than those given a dummy pill.

There are two types of this valuable nutrient: **retinol** which comes from animal produce such as fish liver oils, liver, eggs and butter; and the precursor to vitamin A called **beta carotene** which is found in green- and orange-coloured plant produce such as carrots, oranges and apricots. Beta carotene is converted into vitamin A as it is needed. Any beta carotene left over is used as an antioxidant within the body. This means that it controls free radicals, destructive particles that form inside the body. Because free radicals destroy skin cells and protein fibres within the skin they are the number one cause of facial lines. Eating a diet rich in the antioxidant beta carotene is therefore one of the most effective ways we have in wiping out wrinkles. Many important studies have shown that a high intake of beta carotene leads to low levels of cancer (2). So important are these findings that in 1991 the British Government put almost £2 million of funding into a research project that aims to pinpoint the precise action of antioxidant vitamins.

Beta carotene also protects the skin from sun damage and may be given as a treatment for sun-induced skin itching and swelling. In addition, high doses of beta carotene have a small but significant effect in lengthening the amount of time we can spend in the sun before developing sunburn, (3) an increasingly important factor as the earth's ozone layer continues to diminish.

THE BEAUTIFYING Bs

There are about a dozen **B vitamins** and they all play key roles in safeguarding our appearance. B vitamins occur naturally in unprocessed cereals, brewer's yeast, brown rice, leafy vegetables, meat and fish. Low levels of **vitamin B2** (riboflavin) cause cracked lips, skin rashes and lead to wrinkles and greasy hair. **Vitamin B3** (niacin) helps the body to break down fats and a deficiency is called *pellagra*, literally meaning 'rough skin'. **Vitamin B6** (pyridoxine) regulates the nervous system, combats skin inflammations and maintains healthy teeth and gums. Low levels of B6 can lead to dermatitis-like skin conditions. **Vitamin B9** (folic acid) comes mainly from leafy, green vegetables and prevents dark skin pigmentation. It is also vitally important to prevent neurological birth defects including spina bifida, so it is essential for every pregnant woman.

The only vitamin to contain a mineral element (cobalt) is **vitamin B12** and this is necessary to prevent nervous diseases and anaemia. This vitamin mainly comes from offal meats, oily fish, eggs, alfalfa sprouts and seaweeds and is needed to make new blood cells. Low levels result in a pale, grey or yellow complexion and hair loss.

Other members of the B vitamin family include **pantothenic acid** which has been shown to prevent hair greying and skin ageing; **biotin** which guards against dermatitis and lastly **choline** which assists healthy muscle and skin tissue functions.

C IS FOR COLLAGEN

Probably the best known nutrient of all, **vitamin C**, is also one of our most important. Amongst vitamin C's many functions is the ability to repair and maintain healthy skin by making the protein called collagen that supports the skin. Vitamin C is also an antioxidant and neutralises the harmful effects of free radicals that cause cell damage and premature ageing. These damaging elements form in the lower levels of the skin and lead to many problems, including wrinkles, and the brown pigmentation marks known as liver spots.

Vitamin C is also a powerful healer and can help all kinds of skin lesions, from mouth ulcers and cold sores to burns and grazes. Although vitamin C is plentiful in fresh fruit and vegetables it is easily destroyed by cooking, pollution, stress and by drinking alcohol. Smoking a single cigarette also knocks out the entire quota of vitamin C found in the average orange.

When a food contains vitamin C it will also provide a group of vitamins called bioflavanoids. Bioflavanoids were originally called vitamin P and are also known as flavones or bioflavanoid complex. They consist of several water-soluble, trace vitamins that cannot be stored in the body. This is why eating a regular supply of fresh foods is important to maintain a constantly high level of water-soluble nutrients such as vitamin C and the bioflavanoids. The better known bioflavanoids include rutin, hesperidin and quercetin and our richest sources are apricots, citrus fruits (only in the skins and pulp), cherries, grapes, green peppers, tomatoes, broccoli and buckwheat. Bioflavanoids are especially important for the skin as they work in tandem with vitamin C in maintaining blood vessels, especially the smaller capillaries, and acting as anti-inflammatory agents.

D IS FOR DAYLIGHT

Vitamin D is unusual because it can be made naturally in the skin simply by exposing it to daylight. It can also be obtained from some foods, notably oily fish such as mackerel or herring. Vitamin D is essential for a strong, healthy complexion and firm skin tone. It also works in conjunction with calcium to improve the strength of teeth and bones.

E – THE ESSENTIAL SKIN SAVER

Another warrior in the war on wrinkles is **vitamin E**, also known as the vitality or virility vitamin. Vitamin E is absolutely vital for looking and feeling good. It is an antioxidant, so it also regulates the oxygen production of cells and prevents damage in the deepest level of the skin by free radicals. In addition, vitamin E repairs cell membranes, helps prevent stretchmarks by encouraging greater skin elasticity and boosts the blood circulation.

The best way to guarantee a good supply of this skin-saving nutrient is to eat wholegrains (especially wheatgerm), eggs and *unrefined* vegetable oils (notably wheatgerm, sunflower and safflower oils). However, vitamin E levels are seriously depleted by food refining; cornflakes lose 95 per cent, shredded wheat 90 per cent and puffed rice 80 per cent. The vitamin E content of all vegetables also depends on the storage time. Frozen chips lose 68 per cent of their vitamin E after just one month (as well as most of their vitamin C). Low levels of vitamin E can be a health risk and may increase the likelihood of developing cancer (**4**).

Even if we eat plenty of vitamin-E enriched foods, there are several other factors that may interfere with its absorption. It can be inhibited by oestrogen contained in the contraceptive pill and in hormone replacement therapy, for example. Women taking these drugs should seriously consider adding a daily supplement of vitamin E to their diet. Dr Leonard Mervyn, who has researched many of the medicinal properties of vitamin E, has also discovered another problem with its absorption. Iron is known to deplete vitamin E levels, but there are several types of iron in our diets, including ferric iron which destroys vitamin E and ferrous iron which does not. Iron must be in the ferrous form in order to be absorbed by the body, which is why most supplements contain this version. However, it is incredible but true that the iron added to the devitalised, white flour used in the commercial bread-making can be in the form of ferric salts. Because these are barely absorbed by the body they do not contribute to our iron supplies and, worse still, they can block our absorption of any remaining vitamin E.

The Mighty Minerals

Minerals are another group of essential nutrients that the body needs to sustain life. One of the most critical is **calcium**, required from infancy to build and maintain a strong set of teeth and bones. Calcium also combines with vitamin D to go towards creating healthy muscle and nerve tissues. Calcium is widely available in dairy products (skimmed milk contains slightly more than full-fat milk), nuts, seeds (especially sesame seeds), pulses and many vegetables. The problem with getting enough calcium lies not just in its availability, but in its rate of absorption by the body. Only 20–30 per cent of all calcium eaten is actually absorbed and put to good use. For example, without adequate vitamin D supplies, calcium cannot be absorbed. Also, phytates present in wheatbran tend to bind with calcium, making it difficult for the body to use. Phosphorus also prevents its absorption which is why we should avoid fizzy drinks such as lemonade and cola which are high in phosphates.

Another substance that interferes with the absorption of calcium is lactose, a milk sugar, which must be digested before calcium can be used. Some people cannot digest this milk sugar because they lack the lactose-digesting enzyme called lactase and studies suggest that for some people levels of this enzyme can fall from around the age of four. About 10 per cent are recognised as lactose intolerant to some degree but this figure rises steeply to 80 per cent amongst the African, Indian, Middle and Far Eastern nationalities. Signs of cow's milk intolerance include a blocked nose, rhinitis or runny nose, catarrh, flatulence and diarrhoea. Cottage cheese and yoghurt contain only small amounts of lactose and do not present quite the same problem as cow's milk.

However, all dairy products tend to be mucus-forming and although this is recognised by many doctors it cannot be scientifically explained so is best expressed in naturopathic terms. Naturopaths use natural remedies to treat the body as a whole, not just an isolated symptom. They usually ask patients to avoid dairy products because they create mucus within the body. This occurs not only in those who are lactose intolerant, but in all of us to some extent as our system finds it difficult to break down the complete proteins contained in dairy products. This is probably because the purpose of cow's milk is to fatten calves quickly, not feed humans. Naturopathic principles maintain that as the human body is not designed to digest cow's milk it places a strain on our internal organs, notably the liver, where it acts as an irritant in the system. One of the body's responses to this is to produce mucus, in much the same way as mucus is formed in the nose as a result of dust particles and other noxious substances. This additional mucus is then spread throughout the body making the gut sluggish and contributing to sinusitis, upper respiratory tract problems, coughs and colds. Thirty years ago, the American doctor Robert Gray, who spent many years studying autopsies, reported that milk and dairy produce slow down the transit time of food in the bowel by forming mucus that sticks to the walls of the digestive tract. Dr Gray was a pioneer of the de-tox diet designed to help the body cleanse itself from within. His book *The*

Colon Health Handbook (no longer in print), describes how the colon gradually becomes impacted with waste material as the foods we eat encourage it to build up within the system.

Returning to how we can best make sure we eat sufficient calcium rich foods, the most valuable sources of calcium are:— Gruyère, Cheddar and mozzarella cheeses, plain yoghurt, goat's cheese, sardines, whitebait and sprats (so long as you eat their bones too), skimmed milk, almonds, butter, sesame seeds, caviar, shrimps, kale, pulses, parsley, tofu, chick peas, watercress, dried figs and apricots, scallops, root vegetables, cabbage, broccoli and oatmeal. Calcium-enriched soya milk is another valuable source.

Other lesser known, but equally important, minerals for maintaining good looks are **potassium** and **magnesium**. Low levels of potassium lead to water retention, bloating, headaches and depression. To avoid these symptoms, eat plenty of potassium-rich foods such as bananas, wheatgerm, asparagus, sprouts, mushrooms and drink fresh orange juice. However, potassium must also be balanced with low levels of sodium (salt) to function effectively. Magnesium is found mostly in whole grains, nuts and seafood and primarily guards against skin disorders and hormonal disturbances such as PMT and stress.

ESSENTIAL TRACE ELEMENTS

These nutrients are needed in smaller quantities than the mighty minerals but are nonetheless essential for optimum health and well-being.

Iodine is best known for regulating the thyroid gland that produces the hormone thyroxine. This important substance controls our metabolism and affects energy levels and weight loss or gain. Those who feel constantly tired, irritable or who find dieting a battle may simply not be getting enough iodine in their diet. The richest sources are seafood, fish and kelp or seaweed – one reason why several seaweed recipes have been included in this book.

Iron is another important trace element and despite the fact that Britain is one of the wealthiest countries in the world, iron deficiency (anaemia) is a widespread national problem. Women are particularly susceptible to iron deficiency because of their monthly blood loss and those with heavy periods would almost certainly benefit from a daily iron supplement. One study found that, on average, women between the ages of nineteen and fifty receive about a third less iron than is recommended (**5**). A more recent survey by the Department of Health found that a staggering figure of 90 per cent of teenage girls may be significantly iron deficient. Iron is the most important part of haemoglobin, the red blood pigment that carries fresh oxygen supplies to every cell in the body. It is also an essential part of the connective tissue that supports the skin. Iron deficiency shows up as dull, ashen skin, pale inner eyelids, spots, skin rashes and weak nails.

Iron is found in meat and many vegetables but modern farming practices have depleted our supplies. Chemical fertilisers in the soil bind with iron so that it cannot be taken up by the plant. If the soil is over-fertilised plants become iron deficient and this deficiency continues up the food chain. Cattle or sheep fed on low-iron plant food develop anaemia and as a result human meat supplies are also greatly reduced. Iron absorption is another problem and although it is available in many foods such as offal, egg yolk, shellfish, dried apricots, pulses and green leafy vegetables, its absorption is inhibited by many factors including phytates in wheatbran. So watch the amount of wheat-based products in your diet, such as bread and pasta. Drinking a cup of tea or coffee just after a meal also knocks out about a third of all iron supplied. On the other hand eating a food containing vitamin C will enhance your absorption. For example, a glass of freshly squeezed orange juice supplies the body with enough vitamin C to double iron absorption. Eating raw vegetables with, say, a meat or egg dish also increases the amount of iron available.

The most valuable sources of iron are: liver, fish, soya beans, baked beans, corn, pulses, spinach, rice, wholewheat bread, dried fruit, millet, nuts, blackstrap molasses, pumpkin seeds and green leafy vegetables.

Manganese is a lesser known trace element but plays a vital role in building bones, cartilage and the connective tissue that supports the skin. Manganese also contributes to the protective coating around cells that protects them from bacteria and invading viruses. Many serious disorders have been associated with low levels of manganese, including arthritis, diabetes and heart disease. The best way to ensure an adequate daily dose is to eat plenty of wholegrains (organically grown are best as manganese is destroyed by pesticides), green leafy vegetables and try growing your own alfalfa sprouts.

Selenium is another trace element that has suffered at the hands of modern farming methods. Usually taken up from the soil by growing grains, the level of selenium in our diet has been falling steadily since the advent of chemical fertilisers. Selenium is important for maintaining strong, healthy skin tissues and for preventing hair loss. It works in conjunction with vitamin E and is another antioxidant nutrient capable of scavenging free radicals. The best sources are: organically grown wholegrains, brewer's yeast, avocados, offal, fish and shellfish.

Zinc is the last trace element mentioned, although it is one of the most precious for a clear, healthy complexion. As much as 20 per cent of the body's total zinc supply can be found in the skin and a zinc deficiency often shows up with skin problems such as spots, flaky skin and rashes. Teenage acne has also been linked to low levels of zinc in the diet and small white spots on the nail are another sign that you may be low in this important nutrient. Zinc promotes healing within the body, strengthens the elastin and collagen fibres that support the skin, helps prevent stretchmarks and improves the skin's texture and tone. Zinc is also valuable for improving vision and contributes to clear, shining eyes. Despite its importance, zinc levels in Britain are recognised as falling significantly short of the US and World Health Organisation (WHO) recommended levels. As animal produce is richest in zinc, vegetarians may risk a deficiency. The food groups where zinc can be found include meat, nuts, wholegrains and vegetables, but it is quickly depleted by alcohol and other drugs including aspirin and the contraceptive pill. Chemical fertilisers also deplete zinc levels in the soil and therefore any produce grown in it. Bran, coffee and dairy products can also interfere with zinc absorption.

The most valuable sources of zinc are: meat, sesame seeds, Cheddar cheese, almonds, lentils, haricot beans, wholemeal bread, brown rice and other wholegrains.

Sulphur is a little-known trace element that helps create strong, healthy skin. Sulphur is needed to create the protein called keratin that is found in skin cells, finger and toe nails and in our joints. Hair also contains significant quantities of sulphur, with curly hair containing more sulphur than straight hair. Sulphur is found in several other nutrients including some amino acids, the B vitamins thiamine and biotin, and in vitamin D. Our richest food sources of sulphur are shellfish, horseradish, dried peaches, kidney beans and peas.

Silicon, also known as **silica**, is another trace element needed for healthy skin and hair. This is the second most plentiful element on the planet (after oxygen) and makes up a third of the earth's crust. In humans, silicon is a tiny but vital part of all connective tissues, bones and cartilage. It is also thought to play a part in preventing osteoporosis (weakened bones) as it locks calcium and other minerals into the bones. In addition to this, silicon helps to keep our skin and arteries elastic and our hair and nails strong. Unfortunately, modern food processing strips much of the silicon from foods, such as refined flours and rice. However, organically grown produce, including many vegetables, are a rich source of this trace element.

Amino Acids

Amino acids are the unsung heroes that make up every type of protein in our food. About twenty different amino acids have been identified so far and of these nine cannot be made by the human body. So these nine nutrients are termed **essential amino acids** because it is imperative that we obtain them from our diet. Although we only need tiny traces of these nutrients each one plays an important role in maintaining our health and beauty. The following nine essential amino acids are most abundant in meat (especially game, pork and chicken), wheatgerm, oats, eggs and dairy produce (especially cottage and ricotta cheeses).

The nine essential amino acids are:

Cysteine required to absorb selenium and protect the body from pollution. It also contains sulphur which is needed to control blood sugar levels and create collagen.

Isoleucine is needed for healthy haemoglobin production and skin growth. A deficiency in animals induces tremors and muscle twitching. Low levels of isoleucine have been found in anorexia nervosa patients.

Leucine lowers blood sugar levels and promotes rapid healing of skin and bones. Found to be lacking in both drug addicts and alcoholics.

Lysine required to make collagen in the skin and, according to studies carried out at the Brooke Army Medical Center, Texas, it may also help control the herpes simplex virus. High levels are found in nuts and seeds.

Methionine one of the most significant anti-ageing nutrients as it is involved with producing nucleic acid, the regenerative part of collagen. Good sources of methionine include beans, pulses, garlic, onions and eggs.

Phenylalanine helps regulate the thyroid gland and control the skin's natural colouring due to levels of the pigment melanin. Reputed to be an appetite suppressant and painkiller.

Threonine found in high levels in infant blood plasma to protect the immune system. Regulates neurotransmitters in the brain and fights depression. Some studies indicate it may reduce wheat intolerance.

Tryptophan used as a natural sleeping pill as it has tranquillising properties. Tryptophan is broken down into serotonin, a neurotransmitter responsible for sending us to sleep. Low levels have been found in anorexia nervosa sufferers. One of the best sources is peanuts, although these are difficult to digest.

Valine needed to regulate the metabolism and is used to treat depression as it acts as a mild stimulant. Helps prevent neurological disorders (and possibly multiple sclerosis) as it protects the myelin sheath surrounding nerve fibres in the brain and spinal cord. Low levels have been found in anorexia nervosa patients.

Enzymes

The reason why I have included so many raw recipes in this book is due to the importance of enzymes. These nutrients are destroyed by heat and food processing and can only be found in fresh, raw foods. This means that it is absolutely crucial to include at least some fruit and vegetables in our diet that haven't come out of a tin, packet or freezer bag.

Tropical fruits supply us with some of the more unusual enzymes including **bromalin** (from fresh pineapple) which neutralises harmful bacteria and **papain** (from fresh papaya) that has anti-inflammatory and skin-repairing properties. Some enzymes may also have an anti-ageing ability as they assist in strengthening the collagen and elastin proteins that help to keep the skin supple. Enzymes also work with the body's own digestive juices to break down food in the stomach and increase the level of beneficial bacteria needed to keep the colon and intestines healthy. Enzymes protect us against internal microbial upsets and are important for anyone prone to candidiasis (thrush). In fact, all microbial and fungal disorders such as skin rashes or nail infections are thought to be improved by increased enzyme activity.

The Free-Radical Factor

The most important buzz-words to hit the world of health and beauty recently have been the **antioxidants** and the **free radicals**. Free radicals are created in the course of normal cell activity and in tiny amounts can be useful, but too often they get out of hand and wreak havoc within the body. Free radicals are also caused by other factors such as car exhaust fumes, chemicals, cigarette smoke and radiation (e.g. X-rays).

Free radicals have been linked to most degenerative diseases, notably cancer and coronary heart disease. They are also responsible for almost all skin ageing, which is why many skin creams now contain ingredients such as vitamin E which is an antioxidant, or free-radical scavenger.

Other antioxidants which will help limit the damage done by free radicals are vitamin A (in the form of beta carotene only), vitamin C and the trace mineral selenium. One of the principal reasons why the people of other European countries have lower levels of degenerative diseases such as heart disease and arthritis is now thought to be because they eat many more fruit and vegetables containing antioxidants than we do in Britain.

Essential Fatty Acids

This group of nutrients is currently attracting much attention from nutritionists and the medical world. **Essential fatty acids** (EFAs) come from oils and fats and improve the skin by strengthening the delicate membrane that surrounds each cell. The reason why these substances are termed 'essential' is because they are vital for our health – we cannot live without them.

There are two main types of fatty acids – the **saturated** animal fats, and the **polyunsaturated** and **monounsaturated** vegetable oils. Too much saturated fat from animal sources such as meat, cheese, full-fat milk and butter clogs up our insides, blocks the flow of lymph that carries waste matter out of the body and leads to many life-threatening disorders including heart disease. Saturated fats can also disturb the delicate natural balance of blood fats, resulting in the common problems of greasy hair, spots and pimples. On the other hand, the beneficial EFAs from polyunsaturated and monounsaturated vegetable oils are vitally important to protect cells and actually help prevent many disorders including painful arthritis and eczema. The most abundant EFA in the skin is linoleic acid, found in wholegrains, vegetables, nuts and seeds. Skin also contains other essential fatty acids including EPA and DHA which are only obtained from fish oils.

Trials carried out by the research duo George and Mildred Burr in 1929 found that when rats were fed a diet without EFAs their skin became scaly and their fur clogged with dandruff-like flakes. Unfortunately for the rats, this was then followed by chronic hair loss. These characteristics can also be spotted in other species – humans included – who have low levels of these all-important essential fatty acids. During the last sixty years there have been several hundred papers published into the benefits of oils on the skin. Plant oils in particular have been found to improve dry, scaly skin by strengthening cell membranes to prevent moisture loss. The therapeutic benefits of essential fatty acids has been proved conclusively by double-blind clinical trials. The GLA in evening primrose oil can now be prescribed by your

GP for the treatment of atopic eczema, mostly found in young children. Fish oils, such as cod liver oil, have also been found to benefit some sufferers of acne and psoriasis.

Researchers first decided to investigate the powers of fish oils when it was discovered that native Eskimos (who eat a diet naturally high in fish oil) do not suffer from heart disease, diabetes, acne or psoriasis. However, if they emigrate to Canada and adopt a Western-style diet, Eskimos swiftly succumb to these disorders. This indicates that a fundamental change in their diet plays an important part in their health and beauty. In 1981, Dr Robert B. Skinner, a dermatologist in Tennessee, reported that taking just two tablespoons of cod liver oil a day 'significantly improved' the problem of severe skin hardening and scaling in patients with stubborn skin complaints. Many other medical trials have shown the nutrients in oily fish to be effective in improving the condition and appearance of the skin (6).

The essential fatty acids that have such a marked effect on the skin are tremendous beautifiers in other ways, too, as they also strengthen the structure of our hair and nails. They are easily obtained through food and even the simplest step of adding a few drops of an unrefined plant oil such as virgin olive oil or sunflower oil to our diet every day prevents dry skin, strengthens nails and gives the hair a glossy shine.

Are You Getting Enough?

By now you'll appreciate that our foods contain the building blocks for a better appearance; so doesn't the average diet supply enough of the right nutrients? Surely we don't need a special eating plan, right? WRONG. Despite our increased nutritional knowledge the last fifty years have been a disaster for the face and body, foodwise. Rocketing levels of food processing and over-refining have actually decreased our daily intake of fresh, nutrient-rich, wholesome foods and replaced them with more useless junk than ever before. Of course, it's not only our appearance that's at stake here, the fundamentals of good health are also at risk. Even the Government has finally realised the serious impact that our poor diet is making on the nation's health. The long-awaited Government Health Report released in 1991 by the Committee on Aspects of Food Policy (COMA) highlighted many problem areas. Amongst its most forthright facts is the news that we all eat, on average, **at least** twice as much sugar and saturated fat as we should, and consume far too little fibre.

Despite the undeniable link between diet and well-being our food today is almost unrecognisable from the natural balance our bodies are designed to eat. One way to determine what our daily intake should consist of is to look at the anthropological clues in our teeth. Of our optimum thirty-two teeth, four are pointed, canine teeth to tear meat and fish, eight teeth are incisors that are good for biting into crisp fruit and raw vegetables, while the remaining twenty are intended to chew grains. This dental structure roughly represents the proportions of an optimum diet. Our digestive system gives us further evidence that man was mainly meant to eat unprocessed, plant foods, with his long intestinal tract, as opposed to the short intestines of a carnivore. According to anthropologists studying the Bushmen of the Kalahari Desert in southern Africa, the race thought to lead the life that most accurately reflects that of our forebears, our natural diet consists of 20 per cent fat (mostly unsaturated sources from the oils in nuts and seeds) and 45 grams of fibre per day (compared to 15 grams or less in Western diets). Their data also suggest that our vitamin C intake needs to be at least four times higher than is currently consumed. The average Western diet could not be more different from that of our ancestors if it tried. Highly saturated fat, processed starches, sugar, salt and chemical additives fill the modern shopping trolley, so where are the nutrients the body so badly needs? Unfortunately the answer is that in too many cases, they are completely lacking.

Inferior Foods

Avoiding junk food isn't easy in a society that bombards us with advertisements from every billboard and magazine. We aren't even safe in our own homes – just take a look at the foods and other products promoted in a selection of TV commercials shown during the peak-time breaks of a recent James Bond movie: chocolate, beer, chocolate, coffee, refined sunflower oil, cigars, beer, pizza, gravy granules, chocolate, coffee, artificial coffee whitener, beer, chocolate . . . and so it goes on. Perhaps more shocking is the fact that of the £100 million spent on advertising confectionery alone, most of it is targeted towards the under-twelves, as the commerical breaks during an hour of children's television reveals: sugar-coated breakfast cereals, crisps, cola drink, chocolate snack, crisps, artificial orange drink, processed meat product, sugar-coated breakfast cereal, chocolate snack . . . etc., etc. Changes are occasionally made (the cigar ads were recently stubbed out), but until the junk food giants also admit to damaging our health their commercials remain. But are these foods really so dangerous? Well, don't just take my word for it, here's what the World Health Organisation has to say about the link between diet and well-being. 'Epidemiological research demonstrates a close and consistent relationship between an excess of fat and sugar in the diet and the emergence of chronic, non-infectious diseases – including, particularly, coronary heart disease, cerebrovascular disease, cancer, diabetes, gallstones, dental caries, gastrointestinal disorders, and various bone and joint diseases.' Powerful words with a powerful message – ditch the junk foods!

As adults, we can all make informed choices about what we choose to eat. Children are not given this choice. Bombarded with bewitching advertising and peer pressure, it takes time and effort to re-educate your child's bad eating habits. Of course, it is far easier to pack lunch boxes full of crisps and chocolate biscuits, but we owe the next generation more than this. Taking the right dietary steps *now* helps to ensure a child's long-term health as well as to preserve appearance. In a review on diet and acne, senior skin doctor James Rasmussen states that several foods such as those fried, and all sweets and chocolate, have been commonly implicated as causing or aggravating acne (7). While there is no clear medical evidence to support this, some patients also report that tomatoes, citrus fruits and spicy foods may worsen their acne, which is why it is important to find out if you have any food intolerances. It has also been established that the amount of spot-forming oil secreted by the skin in the form of sebum can be altered by the control of chocolate, milk and refined sugar in the diet (7a). So if we are out to improve our health or beauty (let's aim for both) it is worth avoiding some of the common culprits in order to preserve our looks and well-being.

The Seven Deadly Skin Sins

In alphabetical order, these are the villains:

1. ALCOHOL

Alcohol is the nation's favourite drug, and quite apart from the sustained damage it does to our liver, kidneys, stomach and heart, the adverse effects also show up in our skin. Alcohol is absorbed through the stomach and intestines into the bloodstream where it is rapidly distributed throughout the body. It circulates around the entire system, connecting with every cell and even crossing the placental barrier in pregnant women to reach the developing foetus.

Alcohol causes our capillaries to dilate (widen) and the skin to flush. It also dehydrates the body, stripping vital moisture out of our cells and encouraging premature ageing. The more alcohol we drink, the more nutrients are depleted in the body, especially vitamin A, the B vitamins, vitamin C, magnesium, zinc and the essential fatty acids. Alcohol also encourages your body to absorb lead and aluminium.

Hangovers are the most common side-effect of drinking alcohol and are caused by a combination of chronic dehydration and the chemical colouring and flavouring agents found in almost all drinks. Research shows that people who get migraine attacks would do well to avoid wine (8). Other side effects such as the skin rashes that some people experience from drinking even a modest amount of alcohol can be attributed to the additives. One substance found in almost all wine is sulphur dioxide (E220) which is a common cause of superficial skin reactions, although a severe allergy is rare. Red wine tends to produce more allergic reactions than white because the wine is in contact with the compounds contained in grape skins for a longer period of time. These compounds may include traces of chemical pesticides as vines can be applied with up to fourteen applications of herbicides, pesticides and fungicides while growing and the grapes are not generally washed before processing. Unwanted optional extras can also cause problems – the most tragic example was the death of twenty-two Italians in 1986 after methanol was deliberately added to improve a wine. Other illegal additives such as the anti-freeze slipped into Austrian wine in 1984 and the high levels of MIT anti-fungicide residues found more recently in some 1991 Italian vintages of, amongst others, Soave and Pinot Grigio are obviously undesirable and highlight another major problem, that of labelling.

One of the difficulties with alcohol is that we never know exactly *what* we are drinking. As yet, all alcohol is exempt from ingredient listing, even though many brands of lager, cider and liqueurs such as cherry brandy contain coal-tar dyes including tartrazine, and most wine contains sulphites which trigger asthma attacks amongst sufferers as well as urticaria or nettle rash. Keg beers commonly contain ammonia caramel (E150), propylene glycol alginate (E405) and sulphur dioxide. The foaming agents used in brewing beers contain formaldehyde which is a known irritant and most stouts get their dark 'wholesome'-looking colour from chemical colourants. Even low-alcohol and alcohol-free beers contain many additives including the artificial sweetener aspartame which can react badly with isobutanol, a type of alcohol which remains in these beers after the others have been removed. So while the occasional glass of beer or wine (preferably organically produced) is not going to do a great deal of harm, it is better to reserve alcohol only for special occasions.

2. CAFFEINE

Caffeine is another of the most widely used psychoactive drugs in the world. It is a powerful stimulant that jangles our nervous system, destroys vitamins and minerals, and increases the risk of many health problems including high blood pressure, an irregular heartbeat and pancreatic cancer. It can cause insomnia, headaches, irritability, nausea and diarrhoea. According to a 1989 study published in the *American Journal of Public Health*, just three cups of coffee a day trebles the risk to pregnant women of a low-birth weight baby. Caffeine is a highly addictive substance and most of us in Britain freely admit to being caffeine junkies. Giving up our daily fix requires willpower and determination but the rewards are improved skin tone and luminosity. Research carried out in 1990 at the American University of Vermont discovered that coffee drinkers suffer withdrawal symptoms and automatically reach for a cup to top-up their caffeine levels when they experience headaches, fatigue and drowsiness; and that they experience adverse effects after drinking too much. The findings, published in the *Archives of General Psychiatry*, reveal that for some, drinking just four cups a day meets the definition for symptoms of a drug dependency.

Coffee is the most common source of caffeine (around 60 mg per cup) and according to the pioneering nutritional researcher Dr Robert Erdmann, it may also cause serious side-effects within the skin. All coffee, including decaffeinated, contains benzoic acid, which is toxic to the body. As the body is unable to eliminate this directly, the liver uses an amino acid called glycine to convert benzoic acid into the more harmless hippuric acid. While benzoic acid cannot be eliminated by the kidneys, hippuric acid can be excreted and is present in the urine of all coffee drinkers. So how does this affect our skin? Well, every third molecule in the skin protein collagen is glycine, but as the body's priority is to get rid of poisons in the system it diverts glycine from collagen to the liver. This results in the amino acid being used to detoxify the system while leaving our collagen supplies significantly lowered. A former fifteen-cups-a-day man, Dr Erdmann no longer drinks coffee.

While the occasional cup of coffee made from freshly brewed beans is unlikely to hurt, giving up the demon drink is well worthwhile in the long run. Cutting out coffee or tea (which also contains caffeine), completely from day one is difficult and highly likely to cause dizziness and headaches. How serious the symptoms are depend on how badly you are hooked. When I gave up coffee I suffered from a severe headache for several days, so I suggest you cut down gradually. Try blending your regular brew with a little coffee substitute such as yannoh (made from roasted grains) or dandelion coffee. Gradually increase the amount of coffee substitute until after about two weeks you have weaned your system on to a gentler alternative.

Incidentally, decaffeinated coffee is not the perfect answer because in addition to benzoic acid it also contains other stimulants including theobromine and theophylline which disturb sleep patterns. But if you do choose to drink 'decaff', choose a brand which has had its caffeine removed by natural water filtration and not with chemical solvents.

Tea contains lower levels of caffeine so it is not quite so bad but the decaffeinated versions are well worth trying. Aim to switch to a weaker blend of tea and drink fewer, smaller cups. Herb teas are good alternatives and there are many delicious types around. Watch out for the caffeine hidden in fizzy drinks (notably cola), many medications (especially those for colds and flu) and in chocolate. Carob is a less sweet, caffeine-free alternative to chocolate for those who can't resist a sticky snack.

The caffeine count

Average caffeine levels in drinks per fl oz (25 ml)

coffee 18 mg
tea 12–15 mg
cola 3–5 mg

3. CHEMICAL ADDITIVES

Chemical additives are all around us and almost impossible to avoid in refined foods. Most are listed either by chemical name or by an 'E' number prefix, but some are harder to detect. The words 'flavourings' and 'modified starches' often appear on labels but the individual additives belonging to these groups are not mentioned. There are also about 100 'processing aids' such as solvents that do not have to be declared. Unwrapped bread, cakes and sweets are unlabelled, so we have no way of knowing what chemicals they contain. Pesticides are sprayed on almost all fruit, vegetables and grains to kill insects and fungi. These are then absorbed into the foods and cannot be completely washed off or totally removed by peeling. Fertilisers are taken up by the plant through the soil and may leave high nitrate deposits, particularly in root vegetables. Even though nitrates are known carcinogens (a substance that produces cancer) they are also added in the form of preservatives E249–E252 to meats, processed meat products and some cheeses (including certain types of Gouda and Edam).

Chemical additives are recognised as common allergens. Trials at the Hospital for Sick Children at Great Ormond Street found that the coal-tar food dye tartrazine (E102) was the second most common cause of migraine, after cow's milk. Coal-tar food dyes are also associated with severe hyperactivity amongst children and one of the first medics to investigate this connection was Dr Ben Feingold, an American paediatrician, who linked the explosion in the use of chemical additives and preservatives to behavioural disturbances. Tartrazine has also been found to lower levels of zinc in the body and trigger hyperactivity **(9)**. Despite the medical evidence, tartrazine is still added by some manufacturers to orange drinks, so watch out for E102 on the label before you buy. Better still, make your own naturally healthy squash by mixing the juice of a freshly squeezed orange with a little water.

Coal-tar food dyes are potent by-products of the petroleum industry that cause birth defects and cancer in animals, not to mention hyperactivity and behavioural disturbances amongst

39

children. Yet the average child has already munched his or her way through almost 225 g (½ lb) of these chemicals by their twelfth birthday. The UK and Eire has some of the lowest standards for permitted artificial colours in the world. For example, we still allow the use of E107 (yellow) despite the fact that it is banned in sixteen other countries, including America, France and Japan. The most important additives to avoid are the coal-tar dyes, the benzoates and sulphites (two groups of preservatives) and monosodium glutamate. Some additives are harmless, such as ascorbic acid (vitamin C) and natural colours, so it is worth getting to know which are which (see page 210).

4. SALT

Our average daily intake is around 12 g (½ oz) per day, rising to 20 g (¾ oz) for those who insist on using the salt-cellar with every meal. The World Health Organisation recommends no more than 5 g (⅛ oz) of salt per day. About two-thirds of our salt intake comes from everyday, processed foods. For example, stock cubes and yeast extracts are all high in added salt but can be substituted with a lower salt alternative, although you'll see a little further on that these aren't the complete answer. Excess salt overloads the kidneys and impairs their ability to filter fluids, leading to water retention. Anyone suffering from bags under the eyes or swollen legs and ankles will do well to cut out added salt. Salt is an important factor in the formation of cellulite as it encourages water retention in the skin's fatty tissues. Health-wise we know that salt raises blood pressure, hardens the arteries and upsets our hormonal balance. According to nutritionist Patrick Holford, those who crave salt may be zinc deficient and look to salt to flavour their food. He recommends taking a 15 mg zinc supplement every day for a month while cutting out all salt and salted foods. In his words, 'salt is a pickler and you are the pickle'. Salt occurs naturally in the majority of foods and we really don't need any extra.

As a result of the bad press salt has received over the years there are now many low-salt and salt-free substitutes on the market. However, there are two main problems with these.

Firstly, they usually contain potassium chloride to replace the sodium chloride in salt, and adding too much potassium to our diet disturbs the delicate natural mineral balance needed for healthy kidney functioning. In other words, you could end up with similar problems to taking salt. Advice from Professor Swales of Leicester Royal Infirmary is to use only salt substitutes if you really have to, as too much potassium can harm the kidneys. The only way to free ourselves from the salt-cellar is to re-educate our tastebuds and break the habit forever. Try flavouring foods with fresh lemon juice, a sprinkle of Parmesan cheese, chopped herbs, spices or mustard instead. A limited amount of highly flavoured, salt-based seasonings may be used in cooking, such as tamari sauce (made from soya beans) but ban the salt-cellar from the table!

A pinch of salt

1 level teaspoon salt	mg sodium
cooking salt	*500*
tamari sauce	*440*
sea salt	*350*
sodium bicarbonate (baking powder)	*130*
1 g (0.04 ounce) monosodium glutamate	*180*

Hidden salt in foods

	mg sodium
1 portion average Chinese takeaway	*600*
8 oz (225 g) slice of cheese and tomato pizza	*530*
2 tablespoons baked beans	*430*
1 bowl canned soup, on average	*350*
2 pork sausages	*340*
2 tablespoons low-salt baked beans	*200*
1 bowl high-fibre breakfast cereal	*190*

Sea salt substitute

Sea salt contains traces of other minerals such as magnesium and calcium which dilute its sodium content a little. It contains about 70 per cent of the sodium found in refined cooking salt. Sea salt also has a stronger flavour, so you tend to use less of it. If you can't kick the salt habit completely, grind one part sea salt with six parts sesame seeds and sprinkle over foods. If you want to have some in hand store the combination in an air-tight container in the fridge to prevent the oils from the sesame seeds becoming bitter and rancid.

5. SATURATED FAT

Saturated animal fat is easily recognised as it tends to be solid at room temperature, e.g. butter, suet and lard, unlike the healthier liquid polyunsaturated and monounsaturated fats such as sunflower oil and olive oil. Saturated fat is recognised as one of the main causes of heart disease which causes 40 per cent of all deaths every year. Too much saturated fat also increases your risk of cancer, notably of the breast and colon. The good news is that cutting down on saturated fat reduces the death toll. In America, where the advice to eat less saturated fat and salt has been taken seriously, there has been a fall of 53 per cent in deaths from coronary heart disease over the past twenty years. In Britain, we have so far been slower to change our eating habits and our death toll has dropped by only 9 per cent on average. To get this into perspective, each year coronary heart disease in Britain causes the loss of over 40 million working days, £1800 million in lost earnings and runs up an annual National Health Service bill of at least £500 million. In terms of blood cholesterol, more than 70 per cent of men and women in Britain have levels above 5.2 mmoL/L (the average target).

While eating too much saturated fat is dangerous in the long run, the short-term ill-effects show up more swiftly in our appearance. Because saturated fat clogs up the arteries and interferes with the body's natural metabolism of blood fats it also encourages cellulite to settle on our hips and thighs. Even small amounts of saturated fat slow down the lymphatic system that removes toxins from the body. The lymphatic system is an extensive network that runs parallel to the arteries, but instead of carrying blood the lymphatic vessels contain a milky-white substance called lymph. This acts as the body's dustmen and clears up cellular debris and other unwanted waste matter. While the circulation has a heart to pump blood around the body, lymph relies on a healthy diet and plenty of exercise to keep it moving. A sluggish lymphatic system is bad news for beauty and leads to dingy-looking skin; spots, pimples and acne; rough patches on upper arms; cellulite or the 'orange peel effect' on buttocks and thighs; greasy hair and scalp disorders; dull, cloudy eyes and bad breath.

Cutting down on saturated fat is much easier than it sounds and the health and beauty benefits are very real. Meat is a major source of animal fat, so trim all visible fat off red meat, choose extra lean mince and switch to lower fat meats such as chicken, turkey and game. Those who eat meat should opt for free-range or organically reared produce where possible to avoid the traces of antibiotics and growth hormones routinely fed to intensively farmed animals. Fish is an excellent low-fat source of protein and the oilier varieties such as mackerel and herring contain beneficial fish oils that help fight heart disease and arthritis. Grilling instead of frying foods cuts down on at least half the fat content and tastes just as good. Don't eat more than three eggs a week as egg yolks are high in cholesterol. Switch to low-fat cottage cheese and use low-fat, live yoghurt instead of high-calorie cream. If you can't resist the cheeseboard, make full-fat cheese a rare, occasional treat to be savoured. Reduce your butter rations and replace butter with olive or sunflower oil when cooking. Avoid margarine and low-fat spreads that contain hardened (hydrogenated) vegetable fats as these have been processed to behave in a similar way to saturated fats, so you're not much better off. Hydrogenated fats have been converted from the natural 'cis' form to 'trans' fatty acids which encourage free radicals and have been implicated in cancer. The harder the margarine, the more it has been hydrogenated. Most health food shops sell unhydrogenated spreads which you can use instead.

6. SMOKING

Tobacco has been popular in Britain since the late 1500s although there has always been a health-conscious lobby against it. King James I was ahead of his time when he said 'smoking is a custom loathsome to the eye, harmful to the brain and the black stinking fumes dangerous to the lungs'. Today the damaging effects of smoking are so well known that repeating them seems like stating the obvious. However, here are the facts in a nutshell: smoking kills one person every five minutes and in the last thirty years the number of women dying from lung cancer has risen four times. Smoking causes one-third of all deaths in middle age. In addition to lung cancer, smokers die of lung disease and cancer of the throat and mouth. Nothing else remotely compares with the death toll cigarettes cause. Statistically, out of 1000 young people six will die on the roads and 300 from smoking. About 25 per cent of all coronary heart disease deaths are also due to smoking.

Cigarettes contain nicotine and generate sixteen cancer-causing substances including cadmium, lead, benzopyrene and carbon monoxide. Cigarettes are notoriously hard to give up and nicotine is reputedly more addictive than heroin. Hopefully, you don't smoke, but living or working with a smoker has its own health hazards. Smoking (including passive smoking) generates free radicals, starves healthy blood cells of oxygen and destroys vitamin C. As this book is mainly about beauty you may also like to know that studies in the US show that smoking half a packet of cigarettes a day for just two years doubles your number of premature wrinkles. This is due to the increase in free radicals and the reduction in oxygen supplied to skin cells. Smoking (including passive smoking) also weakens the structure of collagen and elastin fibres in the skin, making it slack and saggy. The cadmium inhaled while smoking specifically interferes with the production of collagen and weakens the skin from within. According to studies carried out by Dr Karen Burke, Director of Clinical Research at the Wilson Dermatology Clinic in North Carolina in 1990, the differences in the facial skin of cigarette smokers compared with non-smokers is vast. Those who smoke have thinner skin and obvious signs of cell degeneration in the lower dermal layers. Dr Burke's findings also record smokers as having more distended blood capillaries (broken veins), ashen complexions with more wrinkles around the eyes and mouth as well as impaired skin tissue healing. No skin-care regime ever invented can repair the amount of damage done to the face and body by smoking.

7. SUGAR

Both brown and white sugar supply calories and absolutely no nourishment. They contain only 'empty' calories and as most of us are concerned about our weight, these are the very last thing we need. Sugar has also been linked to lowered immunity, diabetes and skin disorders such as acne. Too much sugar makes us fat which leads in turn to a much greater risk of high blood pressure, strokes and heart disease. Britain's leading obesity expert, Professor John Garrow at St Bartholomew's Hospital Medical School, London is convinced that it is the unusual way in which sugar is metabolised that is particularly important in its link with obesity, making it more important than previously thought. Other academics to take a stand against sugar include Professor John Yudkin at The University of London, author of the book that pulled no punches entitled *Pure, White and Deadly: The Problem of Sugar* (no longer in print). One area of Professor Yudkin's research includes kidney problems and he has shown that the effects of feeding sugar are first seen in the increased excretion of the enzyme NAG which is seen as an early sign of kidney damage. In humans this can be seen after just two or three weeks on a high-sugar diet and Professor Yudkin points out that the average person's intake of sugar is 1 kg (2 lb) per week, even though there is no requirement for sugar in our diet at all.

The link between sugars and tooth decay is strong and unequivocal. Sugar rots teeth by producing the acid that feeds the bacteria on the surface of tooth enamel. According to the Government health report *Dietary Sugars and Human Disease* published in 1989, 'extensive evidence suggests that sugars are the most important dietary factor in the cause of dental caries'. Tooth decay costs the National Health Service around £20 million a year to treat children's teeth alone. Another horrifying statistic reveals that in 1988 over 84 000 young people in Britain under the age of thirty-four had no natural teeth at all. If this hasn't put you off the stuff altogether, Government guidelines recommend that our daily intake of sugar should not exceed 10 per cent of our total calories, but even this level can be hard to comply with.

Sweet snacks are big business in Britain. During 1990 we spent a staggering £4785 Billion on biscuits, chocolate and confectionery alone. This compares to only £1887 billion spent on fresh fruit – and we all know which will do more good. Sugar dominates these 'foods' because it combines easily with hardened, saturated fats to make highly profitable products. This is why so many chocolate snacks are advertised. What the manufactures fail to point out is that eating sweet, high-fat snacks encourages obesity and rotten teeth.

Consuming less sugar is not only about cutting out sweets though, and it is less straightforward than it sounds. About two-thirds of the sugar we eat is hidden in manufactured foods and is hard to detect without taking a magnifier to the label. Sugar is especially prevalent in processed foods aimed at children, such as sugar- or honey-coated breakfast cereals. As an example, cornflakes contain 8 per cent sugar and when you eat a 'sugar-frosted' cereal your intake increases to a massive 40 per cent sugar. These types of cereals have been specifically targeted by the Health Education Authority as products that we should avoid buying. Less obvious sources of sugar include cola drinks – the equivalent of 8–14 sugar cubes per can – and even savoury foods such as tomato ketchup, tinned soups and most baked beans. Watch out for sugar that is confusingly listed under a different name: sucrose, glucose, dextrose, fructose, maltose, honey, raw syrup, cane and muscovado sugar, molasses and concentrated fruit juice are all forms of sugar.

Sugar substitutes

Those with an impossibly sweet tooth can wean themselves off the white stuff with **limited** use of these alternatives:

Honey *often advocated as the ideal sweetener, honey has a slight advantage over refined sugar. It is a combination of fructose and glucose with traces of enzymes, minerals and vitamins. Honey is therefore a complex carbohydrate and classified as a food, while refined sugar (sucrose) is a simple carbohydrate and is not. However, it is worth noting that bears who plunder the hives of honey bees are the only animals in nature with decayed teeth.*

Fructose *a sugar found in fruits, its chemical composition is easier for the body to break down as the pancreas does not need to release large charges of insulin in order to metabolise it. This places less strain on the system and makes it safe for some diabetics. Fructose is almost twice as sweet as refined sugar so in theory you should use half as much.*

Molasses *a by-product of sugar refining and useful instead of treacle. 'Blackstrap' molasses has had most of the sugar removed and retains the most nutrients, including high levels of iron. 'Barbados' or 'light' molasses has a higher sugar content and fewer nutrients.*

If sugar is so bad for us are artificial sweeteners the alternative? Sadly the answer is no, as a quick look at their contents reveals. The formula for one well-known brand reads like the label on a chemistry set: sodium bicarbonate, trisodium citrate, saccharin, sodium carbonate, glycine and monosodium glutamate. Many medics believe that adding a daily dose of chemicals to our diet is potentially dangerous. Worse still, substances such as saccharin are known to be carcinogenic and in the United States, products containing saccharin are labelled with this direct message *Use of this product may be hazardous to your health. This product contains saccharin which has been determined to cause cancer in laboratory animals.* You can't get labelling much clearer than that.

NUTRITION NIGHTMARES

Despite our affluence, British food is amongst the worst in the world and we are suffering for it. The nutrition scientist Dr Linus Pauling, who has won the Nobel Prize on two occasions, states, 'doctors claim that the ordinary diet will give you all the vitamins you need – this is not true – we do not get the amounts needed in the average diet which does not contain all the nutrients we need for good health'. Some argue that the answer is to take a multi-vitamin and mineral pill every day, but why should we have to pay *twice* for our nutrients? Besides, most supplements contain inferior synthetic substitutes in the wrong proportions to the body's needs. The vitamins Dr Pauling is saying we may not be getting enough of are simply the basic elements of fresh foods, so why should getting back to a wholesome, naturally nutritious diet be such a struggle? Why do we have to search out many of the rudimentary ingredients for an energy-enriching diet in a 'health food' shop? Why can't we simply nip into the local supermarket for our unrefined oils, unhydrogenated margarine, raw buck-wheat and brown rice flour? On a brighter note, many super-markets increasingly stock wholegrains, organically grown and conservation-grade produce, free-range meat reared without growth hormones and antibiotics, low-fat live yoghurt, soya pro-ducts, herb teas, fresh herbs and spices. Clearly supermarkets respond to the law of supply and demand, so if customers contact their local branch manager with a list of regularly requested items these should eventually find their way on to the shelves. But the general reaction to the consumer's call for healthier foods is not nearly as widespread as it should be and the reason for this is because profits are put first. As ardent food campaigner Geoffrey Cannon points out in his book *The Politics of Food*, 'a potato is a small potato. Better is a chip. Better still is a crisp. Best of all is a crunchy waffle . . . rolled out with a £2 million advertising spend'.

Although the quality of some foods is improving the main trend continues away from fresh produce. Each year sees new 'advances' in food technology that has already introduced us to the delights of pesticides, fertilisers and fungicides, chemical colourants, flavours and preservatives and, most recently, food irradiation. The implications of these so-called advancements can be serious for anyone concerned with his or her well-being. For example, Dr John Hunter, a specialist in food allergies at Addenbrooke's hospital, Cambridge reports that about one-fifth of his patients react badly to food additives. Food irradiation is another controversial process introduced solely to suit the convenience of manufacturers by prolonging the shelf life. The method of irradiating foods involves zapping food with nuclear waste at a literally lethal dose of radiation. Irradiating food acts on all the cells within it, destroying their vitamin content and producing destructive free radicals. As free radicals have been implicated in just about every degenerative disease including cancer, it is probably not that sensible to use a process known to encourage them.

The bottom line with all kinds of food processing must be the question 'do these techniques adversely affect the way we look or feel?' Increasingly, health experts believe that they do. The 1990 report by a World Health Organisation study group into diet, nutrition and the prevention of chronic diseases cites the radical changes in food production, processing, storage and distribution, added to modern marketing techniques, that have led to enormous changes in our daily diet. For example, our saturated fat and sugar consumption has increased five to ten times in the past two hundred years, while our intake of complex carbohydrates such as cereal grains has dramatically decreased. The WHO report states bluntly 'changes in dietary habits towards the "affluent" diet that prevail in many developed countries have been followed by increases in the incidence of various chronic diseases of middle and later life'. So while convenience foods have become big business for the powerful food manufacturing giants, they don't do much to create the body beautiful. But the good news is that by following the simple guidelines of eating more wholegrains, fruits, vegetables, oils and herbs you **can** improve your health **and** your looks. This book is your key to the hidden benefits found in every kitchen cupboard. Over the next few chapters you will see that many foods have unique properties – and realise that it really is possible to eat yourself beautiful!

The De-Tox

WHY DE-TOXIFY?

De-toxifying is no longer confined to the cold-turkey drug or alcohol withdrawal but is a foolproof way of ridding the body of all unwanted waste matter. De-toxifying the system is a fast and highly efficient way of thoroughly cleansing the body of a potentially harmful build-up of toxins and pollutants accumulated by modern living. Originally developed by Hippocrates in about 300 BC it is still the safest and most effective way of breaking bad eating habits and restoring high energy levels.

The concept of toxicity within the body is easily shot down by sceptics, yet it remains widely recognised by complementary therapists and valued by those who have actually tried it. The 'toxins' generally referred to are the by-products of normal metabolic processes which accumulate within the system. If there is insufficient opportunity for these to be excreted by the kidneys, bladder and bowel in the normal way, they can stockpile within the system. An example is lactic acid, which must be excreted by the body. If the system is under strain because of a poor diet or stress, it may build up in the joints causing aching and stiffness. This is one reason why a de-tox diet often sees outstanding results when used as a more specific treatment for arthritis. Other so-called toxins are simply the by-products of stress, for example, powerful chemicals like adrenalin that need to be broken down and eliminated by organs such as the liver. If we do not give our body a break from time to time to allow it to 'de-toxify', the entire system is placed under strain and eventually some organ will be adversely affected.

In essence, a de-tox diet gives the body a chance to deal with the waste matter that it otherwise stores in dealing, day in, day out, with the burden of a modern diet. A de-tox diet is so effective at getting rid of toxins that it is widely recognised as an important part in the successful removal of the cellulite that settles on hips and thighs. Liz Hodgkinson, author of *How To Banish Cellulite Forever* (Grafton), maintains that a de-tox regime is essential to cleanse the system from the inside. Her extensive research points to a diet rich in raw fruits and wholegrains as the best way to shift the debris that the body stores in the form of cellulite on our thighs. This notion of internal cleansing is accepted by many medics, including Dr Paul Stillman, a practising GP with a strong interest in holistic healthcare. Dr Stillman is also certain that a low-fat, high-fibre de-tox diet is the chief component for clearing cellulite. In naturopathic and ayurvedic medicines (both of which treat the body as a whole) skin is seen as the third kidney and is referred to as 'the great eliminator'. Certainly we must not forget that the skin is an important eliminative organ, excreting waste matter through perspiration and, to a lesser extent, its own natural oil or sebum. Our skin is an accurate reflection of our internal body chemistry and many of its disorders may be seen as an indication that the body is having internal difficulties.

The principle of de-toxifying is the key that unlocks the body's own natural vitality by ridding the body of the toxins that clog the system and keep it under constant strain. Common ailments can occur when the body becomes overloaded with the substances that the body cannot process. Symptoms of stress, allergies, headaches and skin rashes can all be attributed to internal imbalance. Signs that your system is approaching overload include a lowered resistance to viruses, nervous tension, irritability and cold hands or feet as the metabolism slows down. A de-tox is also the perfect answer for those who simply feel they need an instant tonic or brief rest to recharge their batteries.

HOW TO DE-TOX

All de-tox programmes begin with a period of fasting. Oriental medicine has used fasting as an initial treatment for illness for thousands of years and it is extremely effective. The body takes its cue from nature and it is common to lose our appetite when we are unwell. This is a natural sign that we need a break from food to begin the healing process. Fasting is commonly used in association with several natural therapies, although it is more widespread in other European countries, including France and Germany. One of the many naturopaths in favour of fasting is

Michael Skipwith, senior lecturer at the European School of Osteopathy in Maidstone. He has spent several years working with one of the world's foremost naturopaths, Kenneth Jaffrey, on Magnetic Island, off the coast of Queensland, Australia. Here, Michael had first-hand evidence of extended fasting (for between thirty to forty days) producing remarkable results, even with terminally ill cancer patients. However, he is quick to stress that extended fasting with a view to treating any illness should only be carried out under qualified supervision. From a more general point of view though, Michael says, 'there are no two ways about it, fasting is one of the most useful therapeutic tools to give the human body a rest and help offload toxins. The key is to keep fluid intake up during a fast and only undertake it when you can rest. If possible, be in a relaxing environment with fresh air in abundance.'

THE DE-TOX WEEKEND

The de-tox fast I would encourage you to start with before going on to eat yourself beautiful is far less frightening than it sounds and has been devised to fit into a single weekend. Of course, any two-day period will do, but the weekend is probably when you can allow yourself adequate rest. The first stage is to go without food for a twenty-four-hour period. The easiest time to do this is from 7 pm on the Friday evening after a light supper (such as vegetable soup or a salad) until 7 pm the following day. During your fast you are allowed to (and should) drink as much water as you like (filtered or bottled water is best as it contains fewer contaminants such as chlorine, aluminium and nitrates). Do not drink any other liquid as this may interfere with the de-toxifying process. Some find fasting for a day easier than others and this largely depends on your level of inner health. Generally speaking, the healthier you are the easier it is. So if this is your first fast, choose a time when you have the fewest commitments and can let the body fully relax. It is not sensible to fast when you are under pressure at work or when you have a string of social functions where you are expected to eat or drink. After the first day of fasting it is important to re-introduce foods slowly and carefully.

Break your fast on the Saturday evening with a single variety of fruit. Michael Skipwith suggests a few slices of papaya as this contains the enzyme *papain* which aids the digestion. Apples, pears, grapes and melons are also good choices, but whichever fruit you choose you should only eat this variety for your first meal. On Sunday you may eat raw fruits and salad vegetables, still keep your intake of water high by drinking at least six large glasses. By Monday you will be ready to add more foods, such as nuts, seeds, a few well-cooked grains and vegetable broths. However, you should avoid rich, processed produce, heavy sauces and dressings. By day four you will be feeling refreshed and invigorated and your system will be ready to start the healthy eating programme that will keep you looking good for the rest of your life.

QUESTIONS AND ANSWERS

Do I have to de-tox?

No, but the results will be far better if you do! Unless you give the body a chance to get rid of the harmful substances it has accumulated you cannot hope to achieve inner health and outer beauty. However, if you really can't face going without food for twenty-four hours on day one, you can start the programme with the fruits and raw salad vegetables designed for day two.

Are there any side-effects?

Possibly. Depending on the level of internal toxins that are released prior to expulsion you may experience nausea, lethargy and diarrhoea. Some may find these symptoms more severe than others which is why it is wise to plan your days of de-tox carefully. Unfortunately, those addicted to caffeine are highly likely to suffer from severe headaches. However, any side-effects you might experience are temporary and mean that the body is shrugging off the toxins and waste matter it tends to store.

How often can I de-tox?

Once you have cleansed the system it is then up to you to feed it with the right fuel. If you go back to bad eating habits you will need to repeat the de-tox fairly frequently. Those who continue to eat well should not need to repeat the fast. However, some feel so much better and have so much more energy following the de-tox programme that they decide on a regular weekly or monthly twenty-four-hour fast.

YOUR EAT YOURSELF BEAUTIFUL
LIFETIME DIET PLAN

The de-tox

Day one *pure water only, breaking with a single variety of fruit.*

Day two *pure water plus raw fruits and salad vegetables.*

Day three *as Day two, plus nuts, seeds, well-cooked grains and vegetable broths.*

Re-balancing the body

For the following six weeks, follow the guidelines on page 17, avoiding dairy products and wheat wherever possible. The basic principles are:

Eat daily

Wholegrains 2 or more types

Fresh fruit 2 or more varieties

Vegetables 3 or more varieties (in addition to potatoes)

Unrefined oils 1 tablespoonful

Herbs and spices 2 or more types

Maintaining the body beautiful

From six weeks onwards, you can re-introduce dairy products and wheat if they suit you and you may also add approx 100 g (4 oz) lean meat or fish, or one egg to your daily diet (but limit eggs to a maximum of three per week). Otherwise, keep to the same food groups as set out in the guidelines on page 17. Your new-found vitality, higher energy levels and zest for life, combined with glowing good looks, will be all the evidence you need that this really works!

Try to avoid

Alcohol
Caffeine
Chemical additives
Salt
Saturated fat
Smoking
Sugar

GLORIOUS GRAINS

Eat yourself beautiful with at least two types each day
Grains and cereals are fabulous beauty-boosters. All are an amazingly concentrated source of protein, fibre, vitamins and minerals – in fact, everything the body needs for creating vigour and energy. First cultivated about 9000 years ago, wholegrains such as wheat and barley have had a long and important association with our health. Grains have been the staple foods of many civilisations for thousands of years: wheat, oats, barley and rye in Europe; maize in America; quinoa in South America; rice in the East and millet in Africa. Our ancestors' diet consisted of about 70 per cent wholegrain compared to less than 30 per cent of the average modern diet today – and most of this is refined and over-processed. In their natural state, wholegrains are highly nutritious. Rice, for example, is an important source of protein, magnesium and zinc, all of which are needed to built strong skin cells and healthy nails. Wholegrains are an excellent source of many minerals: oatmeal contains plenty of potassium, magnesium, sulphur and iron; rye flour has significant quantities of potassium, calcuim, magnesium and phosphorus while barley is rich in iron, zinc and sulphur.

The Fibre Providers

The fibre content of unprocessed grains is vitally important for providing the bulk that moves waste matter through the bowel quickly. A sluggish or constipated digestive system causes waste matter to clog up our insides and is the main cause of a sallow complexion. A Ministry of Health report issued in 1991 stated that the average British diet is dangerously low in fibre and that this is linked to many health problems in the Western world. Disorders such as low blood pressure, heart disease, poor circulation and even some types of cancer have all been linked to not eating enough fibre. Adding a little extra fibre-rich food to our diet is the fastest way to clean out the system and will maintain a healthy digestion.

Wholegrain breakfast cereals supply about ten times as much fibre as ordinary cornflakes, so a simple switch in cereal can significantly boost our fibre intake. Adding a spoonful of pot barley to soups or eating potatoes with their (scrubbed) skins also make the most of the natural fibre in our foods. But don't assume that eating foods made from processed grains, such as refined white flour, works nearly as well. The problem with refined flour is that the outer fibrous husk or 'germ' of the wholegrain, such as wheat or barley, is stripped away. The grain is then ground into flour which is often bleached to leach further goodness. Refined white flour contains less than a quarter of the vitamin E found in wholemeal flour and has about a fifth of its magnesium and zinc content. Refined flour is not only a poor source of nutrition, it is also remarkably low in fibre.

The Gluten Connection

Although plenty of fibre is a very important part of a balanced diet, good health and good looks also depend on the **type** of fibre we eat. Wheat bran (e. g. in wheat flours) interferes with the absorption of some of our most important nutrients, such as iron, calcium and magnesium, and can irritate the sensitive lining of the intestines. Wheat also contains a high proportion of a sticky protein mixture called gluten which can fill the delicate foldings of the small intestine, making them less able to function effectively. We take our small intestine pretty much for granted, but it is an amazingly complicated and important piece of bio-design. If stretched from end to end our small intestine would measure about 6.1 metres (20 feet). It has an intricate network of tiny folds that allow it to coil into a compact space just below the stomach. Each fold of the small intestine is covered with micro-receptors that absorb the vitamins and minerals from our food and pass them on into the bloodstream. Their total surface area is staggering – if ironed flat these tiny folds would fill the size of a tennis court! If we rely too much on wheat bran for our fibre the excess gluten may literally gum up the works.

Large numbers of us are mildly intolerant to gluten, while others who suffer from coeliac disease can become seriously ill if they eat any at all. Signs of gluten intolerance and symptoms of coeliac disease include diarrhoea, anaemia due to poor iron absorption, tiredness and recurrent mouth ulcers. Gluten can also cause a skin reaction called *dermatitis herpetiformis* which is recognised by an itchy red rash or tiny sore blisters just beneath the surface of the skin. About one in 2000 have been diagnosed as suffering from the extreme form of coeliac disease in the UK, and this figure rises to around one in 200 in some parts of Ireland. Many more may also be suffering the ill effects of gluten in their diets without realising the cause.

Irritable bowel syndrome is just one of the many modern diseases triggered by a lethal mixture of poor diet and stress. Sufferers are usually advised to switch from wheat to gluten-free grains and often find that their symptoms of bloating, severe constipation or diarrhoea disappear. Even the majority who are able to cope with eating wheat are almost certain to notice an improvement in their digestion if they avoid it for a few weeks – especially if they substitute gluten-free grains such as rice, maize and millet. Perhaps we could then save some of the £60 million each year spent on aluminium-based indigestion remedies and chemical laxatives.

Going Gluten-Free

When I first became aware of the problems associated with wheat I was staggered to discover just how much I ate every day. Like most people I started the day with slices of toast, had a sandwich for lunch, biscuits for tea and probably a pasta dish or pizza for supper. Not far off the national average in fact, but very dependent on wheat-based products, and therefore gluten. Giving up gluten, even for a short period of time to assess the beauty benefits, means watching everything you eat and reading every label. Even an ordinary tin of baked beans has been thickened with wheat flour, and gluten crops up endlessly as a cheap filler for sausages, pâtés and pies, as a thickener for sauces and packet soups, and even in fish fingers and tinned meat. Conventional cakes, biscuits, pasta and breakfast cereals are out – but DON'T PANIC! If you find that most of your shopping list disappears, there are very many healthy and tasty alternatives just waiting for you to get to know.

A Guide To Grains

These are some of the glorious grains and cereal products that play such an important part in creating and maintaining the body beautiful. When buying wholegrains, especially wholegrains that retain their outer husk, it is important to choose organically grown varieties to avoid traces of pesticides. Problems related to eating traces of pesticides are probably more common than we are encouraged to believe and wholegrains may contain more than their fair share.

Delicious and nutritious, grains and cereals safely boost our fibre intake and increase our protein and mineral supplies. The two daily servings of these complex carbohydrates also give the body a slow, sustained release of energy throughout the day, regulate blood sugar levels and reduce cravings for sweet and fatty foods. A daily portion of oat bran has even been found to regulate insulin production and be of help to diabetics. Best of all though, these beauty-boosters are inexpensive, quick to cook and are fantastic for slimmers as they fill us up with only a few calories.

HOW TO COOK WHOLEGRAINS

All rice, millet, buckwheat, barley and quinoa can be prepared as follows. The idea is to absorb all the cooking liquid so the grain's nutrients are retained. Adding the cooking water from lightly boiled vegetables gives extra flavour and the goodness from water-soluble vitamins B and C that would otherwise be thrown down the sink. Varying the basics by adding sunflower seeds, onions, or dried fruit or herbs turns a simple side dish into an adventurous main course.

SERVES 2

225 g (8 oz) wholegrain e.g. rice, barley, rye etc.
1 tablespoon olive oil
2–3 times the grain's volume of filtered water or vegetable cooking water
1 tablespoon sunflower seeds (optional)
1 onion, peeled and finely chopped (optional)

All grains must be washed by rinsing them under running tap water in a sieve. In a large saucepan lightly fry the grains in the oil before adding the water. Add the sunflower seeds and finely chopped onion. Cover and bring to the boil, reduce the heat and simmer for 15–30 minutes (depending on the type of grain) until soft.

Barley

Barley comes from the Middle East but travelled west and has been cultivated in Europe for the last 2000 years. Originally used to make a dark, heavy bread in the Middle Ages, it is still one of the main ingredients in bread baking today, although it is mixed with wheat flour to produce a lighter loaf. Unrefined barley has high levels of iron, calcium, potassium and B vitamins (notably folic acid) and it has unusually soothing properties on the stomach, digestive and urinary tracts. Barley water (see *Pot barley* below) is worth trying for the treatment of stomach ulcers, cystitis and constipation, and is also an excellent internal tonic to brighten up dull, sallow skin.

Pearl barley is the smooth, polished barley kernels which have been stripped of their fibrous husk. Although its fibre content is reduced, it retains some calcium, potassium and magnesium and is excellent for thickening soups and adding to stews. Pearl barley takes about 45 minutes to cook and is delicious mixed with rice or other grains.

Pot barley is the unrefined grain and is coated in a thin layer of nutritious barley bran. Pot barley should be soaked overnight before using, but keep the soaking water for cooking as it will contain important vitamins. It takes about an hour to cook pot barley and it is a delicious addition to rice dishes. To make a healthier version of commercial barley water, simply add 1 tablespoonful of pot barley to 600 ml (1 pint) water, bring to the boil, cover and simmer for half an hour. Add freshly squeezed lemon or orange juice and honey to taste. Strain and store in the fridge.

Buckwheat

Buckwheat is a culinary and complexion superstar and is a *must* for the kitchen cupboard. Historically, it has been important in times of famine as it grows from seed to kernel in a little over two months and thrives in the poorest soils. Originally grown in the Far East, buckwheat is a favourite food of the healthy and long-lived Buddhist monks. As part of the *Kaiho-gyo* ritual of prayer for the attainment of higher spiritual powers, the monks undertake a 100-day fast when they eat nothing but buckwheat. The Japanese are also fond of fresh buckwheat noodles called *soba*, which are available ready-made in health food shops. These are eaten chilled with grated horseradish during the hot summer months to cool the body and revive the appetite. During the winter, the Japanese often add buckwheat noodles to hot broths to warm and fortify them.

Despite its name, buckwheat is totally gluten-free and nothing like our common wheat. It actually comes from a small plant with vivid green leaves related to rhubarb and dock. If you look closely at dock you will see that its seeds have the same distinctive triangular shape. A field of buckwheat in bloom is a pretty sight as each plant is topped with tiny yellow and white flowers. From these flower heads emerge the buckwheat seeds that are harvested as soon as they mature and darken in colour. One of the earliest health food references to buckwheat is in a Japanese food dictionary published as far back as 1697 and reads, 'Buckwheat is sweet, contains no poisons, relaxes the nerves, eases irritability and helps to clear out and release old faeces from the stomach and intestines.' These days, our nutritional knowledge of buckwheat's B vitamins, potassium, magnesium and iron is a shade more scientific and we know it to be an excellent low-fat, non-animal source of the eight essential amino acids the body needs to obtain through food. This makes it especially important for vegetarians. Because buckwheat is so fortifying it is highly recommended for athletes and coaches have been known to advise Olympic rowers to eat it.

Buckwheat is also the richest source of an important bioflavonoid called rutin, which strengthens and tones the network of tiny blood vessels in the skin. It is the perfect skin food for those with fragile skins, red surface veins or broken capillaries. Several different types of buckwheat are available from health food shops and they are all nutritious and highly versatile.

Buckwheat groats can be washed and cooked in the same way as rice, or turned into wonderful risottos (see pages 187 and 195). The vitamins and rutin found in buckwheat dissolve easily in water so it is even more important to add the amount of water that will be absorbed during cooking (see page 61). Buckwheat groats are available either plain or in a pre-toasted version called *kasha* for a stronger flavour.

Buckwheat flour is a pale grey, speckled flour famous for making the gourmet pancakes or *blinis* served in traditional Russian cookery with a dab of sour cream and caviar. Buckwheat pancakes are a delicious guilt-free treat (see page 166) that go down well with the kids, especially when spread with a little honey, blackstrap molasses or real maple syrup (i.e. not made from synthetic flavouring). Buckwheat flour can also be used in recipes for baking and to thicken soups and sauces.

Maize

Maize or sweetcorn was brought back to Britain from America by Christopher Columbus in 1492. It had been cultivated in America for thousands of years and can be traced back to Aztec civilisations. It is a versatile, gluten-free grain and can be eaten whole in the form of corn-on-the-cob, served as sweetcorn or ground into cornflour.

Cornflour is a gluten-free thickener for sauces and desserts. Like all flours, it turns rancid unless stored in a cool, dark place and used fairly quickly. It is best bought in a tin to preserve its shelf life.

Polenta is ground maize or cornmeal and is served on the Continent as a side dish or used to make dumplings and porridge. American cornmeal is much finer and goes into cornbread and muffins. Both types are filling and nutritious but don't contain as much fibre as other unprocessed grains.

Millet

When I mentioned millet to a friend of mine she responded by asking me why I ate birdseed, yet millet was once the most important cereal crop in Europe. Millet is the gluten-free seed of a grass native to Asia and despite its fall from favour in Europe it remains a staple ingredient of African, Asian and Russian cooking. One of the great benefits of millet is that it has the same high protein content as wheat but without the sticky gluten that goes with it. Millet is a complete protein; it contains all eight essential amino acids in the right proportions needed by the body. It also contains more iron than other cereals and is a useful source of calcium. Its unusual protein content is reputed to restore hair loss and capsules containing millet protein are sold with wildly extravagant claims. While I can't guarantee hair growth, millet is an exceptionally nutritious grain and very good for children.

Another interesting fact about millet is that it contains silicon, the cleansing and healing mineral salt that the body needs to make collagen. Silicon is very important for shiny hair, strong nails and general skin elasticity, so a serving of millet is an important part of your skin-care routine. Those who find the taste of millet too bland on its own should try mixing it with other grains. It can be cooked as an alternative to rice but 'crack' the tiny seeds first by frying them in a little olive oil. This helps them absorb enough cooking water to become soft. Millet recipes are on pages 192 and 204.

Oats

Native to Scotland, oats have traditionally nourished and fortified the clans, built up their resistance to the colder climate and given them strength to fight their fierce skirmishes. Today oatmeal remains an important ingredient in many traditional Scottish dishes such as oatcakes and haggis. Oats are an important staple food and contain protein, vitamins B and E as well as, perhaps rather surprisingly, the healthy polyunsaturated fats. Oats are also a rich source of calcium that builds strong teeth and bones, in addition to other minerals such as potassium and magnesium.

Today's oats are milled to produce different textures – from finely ground oatmeal to the medium and coarsely ground varieties required for baking and making porridge. Porridge oats are easy to find in the supermarket and are an excellent family breakfast cereal. They are also a good base for healthy snacks such as flapjacks. Although long associated with healthy eating, nutritionists have only recently pin-pointed the benefits of adding oats to the diet. They have discovered that a few spoonfuls of oat bran taken every day can dramatically reduce a high cholesterol count. This is because the unusual fibre in oat bran neutralises the bile acids that would otherwise be converted by the liver into cholesterol. Oat bran has also been shown to regulate blood sugar levels and may even help diabetics as it encourages insulin stability. Special soap and skin creams made from oat bran help heal skin complaints such as eczema, psoriasis and acne, and adding a daily dose of oats to the diet also seems to reduce skin inflammations. The organically grown brands are especially good.

Quinoa

Quinoa (pronounced keenowa) is a tiny, golden grain similar in shape and texture to millet. Unlike most grains, quinoa does not belong to the grass family but is a relative of the garden weed commonly known as 'fat hen'. It has been cultivated since 3000 BC in the South American Andes where ancient Incas called it 'the mother grain' and held it sacred. Since then, quinoa has been hailed by naturopaths as a balancing grain that 'grounds' the body and encourages inner peace. Nutritional science, on the other hand, values this unusual food for its higher protein content than most other grains (around 14 per cent compared to 8 per cent for most rice) and its source of both essential fatty acids and amino acids. Typically, a single serving supplies over 9 g of protein and almost all the amino acids. Quinoa cooks quickly in 10–15 minutes and can be mixed with other grains to improve what even the most meditative must admit to being a fairly bland flavour.

Wheat

Wheat is Britain's most important crop and, not surprisingly, our diet is dominated by it. Over 30,000 varieties are said to be in cultivation but almost all belong to two main species. These are *Triticum aestivum* used for bread baking and a harder wheat called *Triticam durum* used for making pasta and semolina. As mentioned earlier, wheat, and all its products, have a high gluten content. In fact in bread baking it is the gluten which gives a loaf its elasticity.

Couscous is a refined wheat product made from semolina (see below) and is the staple food in North Africa where it is served with hearty fish and lamb stews. It is wonderfully easy to cook – simply pour boiling water over it and simmer for a few minutes until the grains are fluffy and soft. However, some of the wheat's original goodness is lost in its processing and it also lacks fibre.

Cracked wheat or bulgar wheat is another processed wheat product made from broken grains. The most nutritious way to eat cracked wheat is pre-soaked and served in a raw Lebanese salad dish called Tabbouleh (see page 178).

Semolina is the grittiest part of durum wheat, sifted out and made into hardened pasta products such as dried spaghetti and macaroni. Semolina can also be used on its own to make puddings but it is a highly refined product and contains little fibre.

Wholewheat or wheat berries are simply the wholewheat kernel and are the best way to enjoy wheat, despite taking a while to cook (unless you live near a field and ask the farmer for a fresh handful). Dried wheat berries are best soaked overnight to soften their tough outer husk. Then add some more water or vegetable juice and simmer them for about an hour. Well-soaked whole-wheat can also be added to home-made bread or scones and makes an unusual extra for soups and casseroles. Wholewheat is also superb sprouted (see page 77).

Wheatgerm is the inner core of the wheat grain and is nature's richest source of vitamin E. Raw wheatgerm is a good source of protein and very high in iron. It is one of our most important nutrients for healthy, young-looking skin and a packet of wheat-germ in the kitchen is as valuable as a jar of moisturiser in the bathrom. Wheatgerm flakes or toasted wheatgerm can be sprink-led over almost anything to boost its beauty benefits. Try adding a spoonful to soups, sauces, breakfast cereals and even desserts such as stewed apples and apricots or low-fat yoghurt. Wheat-germ is naturally protected from rancidity by its high vitamin E content but should be stored in a sealed tin or jar away from heat and light (in the fridge if you prefer).

Wholemeal flour is made from wholewheat grains and it is a good source of protein and some minerals including potassium, phosphorus, magnesium and calcium. Wholemeal flour is added to many types of pasta including spaghetti to boost its fibre con-tent. Brown wholemeal flour contains added wheat bran, although watch out for those with artificial colouring that simply dye the flour a healthier looking colour. Bread, biscuits and cakes made with wholemeal flour contain more than twice as much fibre and other nutrients than those with white flour, so it is well worth making the switch.

Rice

Rice is another fabulous staple food for families all round the world. Provided it is stored in a cool, dry place rice will last almost indefinitely, so you can safely store several different types to use over a period of many months. There are over 7000 varieties of rice, all of which are inexpensive and easily available in many forms, including organically grown. All types of rice are easily digested and highly unlikely to cause any allergy problems. For these reasons flaked rice is universally recommended as a baby's first solid food when weaning. Puffed rice makes a good breakfast cereal (you can find sugar-free, organically grown varieties in health food shops) and rice cakes are tasty low-calorie snacks. All rices and rice products are gluten-free.

Basmati rice comes from the foothills of the Himalayas and is a fine, long-grain rice. It has a naturally aromatic flavour and is the perfect accompaniment to curries or spicy foods. I find it improves if soaked for at least half an hour to allow the grains to split and soften, but use the soaking water for cooking as some of the rice's important vitamins pass into it. Brown basmati rice contains more fibre and protein than the polished variety and is delicious served on its own or mixed with Italian or brown rice.

Brown rice is the entire rice pellet, including its protective bran coating and is an excellent source of fibre and protein. Brown rice also contains iron, calcium, B vitamins and many essential amino acids, and you wouldn't go far wrong if you ate it every day. In fact, those who follow the ultimate healthy – but fiercely strict – Oriental macrobiotic way of eating insist that 70 per cent of their daily food intake consists of brown rice or similar grains.

Carolina rice or patna rice is most commonly found in packets. It is highly polished, has a bland papery taste and I don't much like it. It was originally eaten unpolished and provided millions of people with a rich natural source of B vitamins. With the advent of food refining, the nutritious husks were lost and a serious disease called beri-beri (caused by vitamin B deficiency) spread throughout the Far East. If you really want to use it, mix it with other brown varieties of rice for additional nutrients, fibre and flavour.

Glutinous rice despite its name contains no gluten at all, but it does have a sticky, glutinous texture. This makes it a popular choice for Japanese and Chinese cooking as the grains clump together and are easier to eat with chopsticks. Naturally sweet, glutinous rice is a good choice for puddings and Chinese cooks use it for baking and confectionery making.

Italian rice is the perfect choice for making risotto as its large, oval shape gives texture to these famous Italian rice dishes. Brown Italian rice is both healthier and tastier.

Wild rice, strictly speaking, is not a rice at all but a seed from an American water grass called *Zizania aquatica*. It has a long, dark brown, elegant shape and a uniquely nutty flavour. It is expensive, but a little goes a long way and a spoonful can be cooked with plain brown rice to turn an ordinary dish into something special. Wild rice stuffing is a traditional accompaniment to poultry and game, and is delicious combined with dried chestnuts or apricots.

Pudding rice has a short, round shape and looks quite different from other varieties. It is highly polished and becomes mushy when cooked, giving us little in the way of fibre. Sweet brown rice is a better choice for making rice puddings.

Sweet brown rice is the perfect choice for the ultimate rice pudding (see Nice Rice Pudding page 208). Sweet and sticky, yet decidedly good for us, it is an essential cooking ingredient.

Rice flour consists of the flour milled from both white and brown rice grains. It has a soft, silky texture favoured by the cosmetic industry for making some types of face powder and talc. It is also a versatile cooking ingredient and can be used alone or mixed with other flours to make cakes and biscuits. Expert cook Sophie Grigson uses a spoonful of rice flour to lighten some of her recipes and substitutes rice flour for two-thirds of the wheat flour when baking cakes in the microwave. It is well worth keeping a jar of it to hand as it deliciously thickens soups, stews and sauces. Rice flour does take slightly longer to cook and soften than ordinary wheat flour though, so allow yourself a bit of extra cooking time or your recipe may taste a bit gritty.

Rye

Rye has a similar composition to wheat but has a low gluten content. Black rye bread made with rye flour is a delicious alternative to your usual loaf and toasts well. Rye crispbread and crackers are also easy to find in the supermarket and make an interesting change to wheat-based varieties. Rye flour can also be mixed with wheat flour for home baking.

Sago

Sago comes in dry granules obtained from the sago palm in the Far East. It is very easily digested, has no allergy problems associated with it and is traditionally used for making milk puddings for invalids. Although bland and lacking in fibre, sago is useful for those on a restricted or gluten-free diet.

Soy Flour

This soft, golden powder is not a true flour because it comes from ground soya beans, but it is gluten-free and a useful source of protein. Soya flour can be added to thicken sauces and soups, as well as for baking.

Tapioca

Tapioca is another unusual but useful addition to the kitchen cupboard. Tapioca is a small pellet made from manioc flour which comes from the tropical *manioc* plant in Central Asia. It can be used as a gluten-free thickener or as the basis of milk pudding.

Beautiful Beans

Beans and pulses such as chick peas and lentils are a good source of protein, minerals, fibre and B vitamins – all essential for strong, supple, clear skin. Lentils in particular are a useful source of iron, although as they contain purines they should be avoided by those suffering from gout. Gout is one form of arthritis in which diet is known to play a part and those with gout need to watch what they eat. This disorder is caused by higher than normal levels of a substance called urate, which is formed from purines in food. In addition to lentils, foods high in purines include yeast extracts, bacon, liver and sardines.

Beans and pulses have been the staple foods for many different civilisations around the world and are now making a timely comeback in Britain. The best way to serve them is combined with wholegrains (e.g. rice or millet) to balance the different essential amino acids in each of these groups of food and thereby maximise their protein content. This is because wholegrains and beans contain different proportions of amino acids and you can ensure you get enough of all eight of the essential amino acids by combining the two types of foods. For example, most grains do not contain the amino acid *lysine*, which is why it is a good idea to eat them with pulses which are rich in *lysine*. Try mixing rice with butter beans, barley or rye with lentils and couscous with a chick pea sauce. Combining wholegrains with nuts and seeds is also a good way to ensure you are getting the right balance of amino acids that the body needs to function healthily. Having made this point about combining cereals and pulses (and introducing nuts and seeds), new research seems to indicate that it isn't vital to eat the different foods at the same meal. It looks as if by eating a range of protein sources during the day the body will use its 'pool' of amino acids to ensure first-class protein availability.

As with the wholegrains, beans are nutritional nourishers which are well worth getting to know as they fill us up with only a few calories. All beans and pulses are a bit tough to digest though and can give us wind, especially if you are not used to eating them. The way to get round this is to cook them with an ingredient that counters flatulence. Macrobiotic cooks add a small piece of dried kombu seaweed or you could throw in a few caraway, coriander, dill or fennel seeds. The Vegetarian Society, which produces an information sheet entitled *Cures for flatulence* also recommends chewing a few dill or caraway seeds after a meal. These ingredients are traditionally used to help break down the substances in beans and pulses that the stomach finds difficult to digest. Even the most exotic types of pulses and beans are now available pre-prepared in tins from supermarkets, although some can lack the subtle flavour of freshly soaked varieties. Buying the dried form and soaking them yourself not only works out cheaper but is also the best way to appreciate their true taste. The snag is that you must remember to allow enough time to soak (if necessary) and cook them before adding them to your recipe.

Preparing Beans and Pulses

All varieties **must** be brought to the boil for at least 10 minutes to neutralise the acids that can cause severe stomach pains, then reduce the contents to a gentle simmer. The following gives a guide to soaking and cooking times, although cooking times will vary slightly depending on the quality of the beans and pulses. After the soaking time discard the soaking water, rinse the beans or pulses under cold water, and then use fresh water to cook them in. Once they are cooked it is better to discard the cooking liquid which will have absorbed sugar-like substances that can be another cause of flatulence.

Aduki beans	No need to soak, cook for 35 minutes.
Black-eyed beans	No need to soak, cook for 35 minutes.
Borlotti beans	Soak overnight in cold water, or for 2 hours in boiling water, cook for 1 hour.
Butter beans	Soak overnight in cold water, cook for 1½ hours.
Chick peas	Soak overnight in cold water, or for 2 hours in boiling water, cook for 4 hours.
Dried peas	More nutritious than split peas. Soak overnight in cold water, or for 2 hours in boiling water, cook for 1½ hours.
Flageolet beans	Soak overnight in cold water, or for 2 hours in boiling water, cook for 1 hour.
Lentils	No need to soak, check and discard any small stones, cook for 30 minutes.
Red kidney beans	Soak overnight in cold water, or for 2 hours in boiling water, cook for 2 hours.
Mung beans	No need to soak, cook for 40 minutes.
Soya beans	Soak overnight in cold water, or for 2 hours in boiling water, cook for 4 hours.

Superb Seeds

ALFALFA SEEDS

Don't let the size of these tiny seeds fool you as they are an amazingly rich source of concentrated goodness. Alfalfa seeds need to be sprouted before using (see page 77) and this releases the valuable energy and nutrients that feed the growing plant. When grown in the wild alfalfa shows remarkable skills of self-preservation and puts down roots up to 30 metres (100 ft) deep. It is highly resistant to pestilence and drought, and is now being cultivated in many Third World countries in an attempt to prevent starvation.

Alfalfa sprouts are best eaten shortly after germination as this is when they contain their highest vitamin and mineral levels. This is usually when the sprouts measure 1–5 cm (½–2 inch) long. Alfalfa contains complete protein with all eight essential amino acids, high vitamin and good mineral levels, and several enzymes to improve digestion. It is a good source of calcium and B vitamins, including the elusive vitamin B12. This nutrient is usually obtained through meat, although other vegetable sources include soya beans, seaweed and an unusual Mexican algae called spirulina. Alfalfa is therefore an important ingredient for vegetarians, vegans and anyone wanting to cut down on meat rations. Alfalfa sprouts are used therapeutically as a tonic, a mild diuretic and intestinal cleanser. When buying alfalfa seeds, or any other seed or grain for sprouting, choose organically grown varieties as these will not be coated with pesticides.

PUMPKIN SEEDS

Pumpkin seeds can improve your sex-life, or so the Hungarians claim and they munch them by the handful! Long linked in folklore to male virility, these dark green seeds contain useful amounts of iron, zinc and calcium, as well as some protein and B vitamins. While no scientific studies have proved their aphrodisiac powers, it has been noted that the Eastern European countries where

pumpkin seeds are eaten regularly have very low rates of pro-
state trouble (a common, middle-aged male disorder). Pumpkin
seeds are a delicious addition to many recipes and give extra
crunch to salads. They are also a tasty raw snack food.

SESAME SEEDS

Sesame seeds are an outstanding source of calcium and a rich
source of protein. They also contain iron and zinc and should defi-
nitely be eaten by vegetarians and vegans who may lack these
important nutrients. The tiny sesame seed also contains plenty of
vitamin E and lecithin, a substance that locks moisture into the
skin and prevents dry skin and signs of premature ageing. In addition, sesame seeds are a particularly good source of one of the
eight essential amino acids called methionine. This is needed for
healthy kidney functioning and a good supply helps prevent
swollen skin tissues and puffiness caused by kidney disorders.
Methionine also contains sulphur which is needed to create the
protein keratin in our hair and nails. Sesame seeds are as versatile as they are nutritious and can be added to almost any
recipe. They may be ground into a thick savory paste called *tahini*
or blended with honey to make a Greek sweetmeat called *halva*.
You can also whizz up a handful in a food processor with a pint of
water to make sesame milk. This is a good base for non-dairy milk
shakes and, if you're feeling really adventurous, can even be
turned into sesame yoghurt or curd cheese.

SUNFLOWER SEEDS

Sunflower seeds are another exceptionally good skin food and
contain generous amounts of protein and amino acids including
methionine. They also have high levels of vitamins, minerals,
fibre and essential fatty acids. The Roman army munched sesame
and sunflower seeds to sustain their strength on long route
marches and in Russia millions have survived famine by eating
virtually nothing but sunflower seeds. These nutritious nuggets
are rich in vitamin E, B vitamins and contain reasonable amounts
of iron, magnesium and zinc. These are the nutrients needed to

increase our resistance to disease and build strong, healthy connective tissue in our cells. Sunflower seeds also contain pectin which helps prevent lead poisoning from car exhausts and removes toxic wastes from the body by combining with them into chemical compounds that allow them to be excreted. Naturally sweet and full of iron, sunflower seeds are a delicious, nutritious snack. They are useful as an extra ingredient in many recipes and can be ground in a coffee grinder and added to a frothy milk shake (see Super Seed Shake page 165), sprinkled whole on salads or added to bread and flapjack mixtures. Almost half the sunflower seed is taken up with polyunsaturates, the beneficial fats that keep our cholesterol levels in check and prevent our arteries from becoming clogged. Sunflower oil is produced from the crushed seeds but loses almost all its nutrients in the refining process. So if using sunflower oil for cooking choose the unrefined versions available from health food shops.

THE SKIN-SAVING SUPER SPROUTS

No praise is too high for these fantastic skin-savers and we can all increase our strength, stamina and sort out many skin problems simply by eating a small amount of sprouted grains and seeds every day. Most grains, beans and seeds can be sprouted to increase their vitamin, mineral and enzyme levels dramatically. Sprouting also releases important amino acids that improve the quality of protein and neutralises the phytates found in grains that impair zinc and calcium absorption. The most successful varieties for sprouting are alfalfa, lentils, mung beans, millet, sunflower seeds and the wholewheat (or wheat berry) grains.

Sprouted foods are also the ultimate in freshly picked, organically grown food and it's so simple to become a D-I-Y kitchen farmer. You can buy special sprouting containers from health food shops but it is just as easy to make your own. All you need is a large jam jar, a clean disposable wiping cloth or piece of muslin and an elastic band. Simply put a handful of pulses or seeds in the bottom of the jar, cover the top of the jar with the cloth and hold firmly in place with the elastic band. Run some cold water into the covered jar, invert it and let the water drain away. Repeat this rinsing several times a day until all the shoots have appeared. Leaving the sprouts on the window sill or under a light encourages them to darken by producing chlorophyll. This is also a good way to increase their magnesium and fibre content.

Sprouts are delicious eaten raw in salads or sprinkled with a little freshly squeezed lemon juice. Top French chefs even stir sprouted wheat grains into soups and sauces, but as their vitamin and amino acids are destroyed by heat they are best eaten raw.

Nutritious Nuts

Nuts, like seeds, are very nourishing and packed with all the nutrient the plant will need in growing. They are rich in vitamin E and many minerals including zinc and iron. Although relatively high in calories, nuts are an excellent protein-packed alternative to high-fat cheese and meat. All nuts should be eaten raw and as fresh as possible as they turn rancid when exposed to heat and light. For this reason it is best to avoid processed or dry-roasted nuts, which are also highly salted. Nuts last longest when stored in an airtight container in the fridge and can also be frozen.

Any type of nut can be turned into a delicious nut butter simply by being mixed in a food processor for a minute or two. Just add a little water or apple juice until you reach the right consistency. Peanut butter not only costs less but is also much fresher made at home, or try a more exotic blend such as cashew and hazelnut or almond butter.

Almonds are a good source of protein and several important minerals including zinc and iron. They also contain the essential fatty acids that keep skin supple and hair shining. Eating a handful of almonds every day, or taking almond oil capsules, is also one of the best ways to strengthen flaky nails and prevent white spots and ridges. Almonds are best eaten straight from the shell or at least bought with their dark skins on. Blanched almonds lose much of their nutritional value and are almost tasteless by comparison. Ground almonds are best bought in small quantities as they go off fairly quickly once opened. Alternatively, grind your own supplies as you need them. Finely ground almonds are useful for thickening sauces, stews and curries, and are delicious mixed with a little *fromage frais* for a healthy dessert. They are also stirred into yoghurt as a good baby food (make sure there are no small pieces that a child could choke on) and can even be blended with water to make almond milk.

Brazils grow on tall forest trees in South America in large pods that contain between twelve and twenty-four nuts. They are another useful source of the essential amino acid methionine. Brazils are best eaten as a fast-food snack or mixed with other types of nuts in salads. Finely pulverised Brazil nuts are an interesting change from ground almonds and also make a delicious nut butter, simply by putting them in a food processor. As they only grow in rainforest conditions, a higher demand might help preserve the Brazilian rainforests.

Cashews are native to America and on the trees they are attached to a fleshy, apple-like fruit. They are a good vegetarian source of the essential amino acid lysine which is more commonly found in animal produce. Cashews are a rich source of protein but also contain a good deal of the unwanted saturated fat that clogs our arteries. For this reason cashews are best kept as an occasional treat. Cashews are a tasty addition to many dishes and a few thrown into an ordinary chicken casserole just before serving give it a gourmet touch. Cashew cream is also a delicious, highly fattening but unusual dairy-free alternative to double cream. Simply blend a handful of cashews in a food processor with a tablespoonful of water and a few drops of vanilla essence.

Chestnuts can be bought fresh in the winter but they are a real fiddle to skin so I buy mine dried. You can also find tinned, whole chestnuts and chestnut purée, but watch out for added salt or sugar. Because they contain less natural oil and more starch than other nuts they are more suitable for cooking. Chestnuts are delicious added to vegetable dishes such as Brussels sprouts or parsnips and their soft, starchy texture is ideal for pâtés and stuffings. Chestnuts are naturally sweet and a healthy ingredient for many puddings and pastries.

Hazelnuts are the lowest in fat of all nuts and are rich in vitamin E, making them a nutritious skin-saving snack. Hazelnut oil is one of the newest additions to the supermarket shelves and is a versatile cooking oil. Try adding a few drops to wholegrain biscuit mixtures or flapjacks for a deliciously nutty taste.

Peanuts are not really nuts at all but belong to the same legume family as the soya bean. They are especially rich in protein, iron, vitamin E and B vitamins (notably folic acid). However, all legumes can be hard to digest and peanuts are no exception. They are best when ground into peanut butter or as a snack eaten fresh from their shells.

Walnuts are grown on trees that are harvested for their timber as well as their nuts. They are high in calcium and have an unusually strong flavour that is perfect for tossing into the classic Waldorf salad along with slices of chopped apple and celery. Walnut oil has been used for centuries to prepare artists' oil paints and is also available for cooking. However, as its structure changes when heated it is best used cold, such as to flavour salad dressings.

Protein Power

All grains and pulses, such as peas, beans and lentils, can be a healthy low-fat substitute for animal protein in everyone's diet. The key is to eat them in the correct combination to complete their protein content. As we have seen, the protein in pulses contain the essential amino acid, lysine, which is not found in grains. When eaten together, however, pulses and grains create a high quality protein which is similar to meat. The main difference is that it is low in fat, cholesterol-free and less expensive. Many animal proteins actually contain more fat than protein. For example an average steak is 20 per cent protein, 80 per cent fat, Cheddar cheese is 25 per cent protein, 75 per cent fat, chicken breast (without skin) is 65 per cent protein, 35 per cent fat, and a fillet of cod is 90 per cent protein, 10 per cent fat. As kidney beans are 25 per cent protein, 5 per cent fat and 70 per cent carbohydrate, they are a healthier source of protein than steak, provided they are combined correctly.

As the body cannot store protein it needs to be supplied on a daily basis. The body seems to use protein most effectively if it is eaten frequently throughout the day. Several smaller meals containing some form of animal or vegetable protein are more easily absorbed than a single blow-out at one sitting.

Good combinations of pulse and grain dishes include
Baked beans on toast
Lentil lasagne
Rice and beans
Pea soup with bread or crackers

Nuts and seeds are also a rich source of vegetable protein. Unlike grains and pulses, however, they also contain high levels of fat in the form of natural oils. Even though the fat found in nuts and seeds is in the healthy unsaturated form, they are high in calories and should be used in moderation. However, nuts and seeds are excellent companions for serving with other vegetable proteins. When eaten with plain cooked rice, grains or pulses, a sprinkling of nuts and/or seeds ensures the dish is a complete serving of protein.

Good combinations of nuts and seeds include
Humus – a dish combining chickpeas with sesame seeds
(recipe on page 174)
Rice risotto served with chopped nuts
Bread or rice cakes spread with nut butter, such as peanut butter
Tofu (soybean curd) dipped in sunflower seeds.

FABULOUS FRUITS

Eat yourself beautiful with at least two varieties each day. Eating a minimum of two varieties of fresh fruit each day is one of the best-kept beauty secrets. Not only is fresh fruit an important source of vitamins, minerals and enzymes, but its high fibre and water content make it the most magnificent internal cleanser. This is because the fibre binds with toxins and impurities in the body so that they can be removed while the water gently flushes them out of the system. Fruit is also fat-free, very low in calories and yet naturally sweet, so it is ideal for those watching their weight. Fresh fruit also plays an important role in protecting our health and well-being and the World Health Organisation recommends that we all aim to eat around two portions of fruit a day. This is about 1.75 kg (4 lb) of fruit a week, compared with our current national average which is closer to 550 g (1¼ lb) according to the 1990 National Food Survey.

The importance of fruit in controlling disease was highlighted as long ago as 1922 when the British surgeon, Robert McCarrison, returned from an expedition to Hunza in north-west Pakistan. As he wrote in the *American Medical Association Jour-*

nal, 'The Hunzakuts have no known incidence of cancer. They have abundant crops of apricots which they use very largely in their food'. This observation endorsed the view of a group of American researchers investigating an anti-cancer substance tagged B-17, which is found in Hunza apricots and other fruit seeds and pips. Scientists in Japan have also succeeded in isolating fruits which contain powerful anti-mutagens that may help to further diminish the cancer threat. Their list of 'good guys' includes pineapples and apples (as well as broccoli, ginger, green pepper and cabbage) which have all been found effective in blocking cancer-promoting cell mutations. While we wait for the elusive cure for cancer, the New York Cancer Research Institute has reported encouraging results with beta carotene supplements (also known as carotene). Beta carotene is found in many yellow, orange and reddish-coloured fruits, along with several other useful vitamins such as vitamins C and E. These three nutrients are known as antioxidants as they repair the damage caused by free radicals resulting from cell oxidation. A diet rich in beta carotene, vitamin C and vitamin E will improve the appearance of the skin by protecting skin cells deep in the lower levels of the dermis and defending against the signs of premature ageing. It is also worth noting that vegetarians who eat far greater quantities of fruit than the national average also enjoy a lower incidence of cancer and heart disease, thought to be the result of a higher intake of these protective elements.

The Enzyme Connection

Fruits are most beneficial when eaten raw as they contain valuable enzymes that trigger a huge range of chemical reactions within the body. Fresh lemon juice contains the enzyme *esterase*, an antiseptic, but like most enzymes it is destroyed by cooking at high temperatures. Enzymes also perish when exposed to air and so fruit is best eaten as soon as it has been cut. Nutrient values also begin to diminish as soon as the fruit has been picked and some fruits, such as oranges, may be stored for many months before reaching the supermarket shelves. Always avoid fruit that looks past its best and ignore any with obvious patches of mould as these microspores may aggravate cases of thrush caused by the *Candida albicans* microbes. Fruit should be firm to the touch and have a fresh aroma which indicates that it is ripe and sweet. One way to be sure that the fruits you are buying are freshly harvested is to choose organically grown produce. Because organic fruits are not sprayed with preserving agents they tend to grow green whiskers if not sold quickly and you are more likely to spot fruit which has been sitting on the shelf for too long.

Sweet Talk

All fruits contain fructose, a natural sugar with the same number of calories as refined sugar but up to 30 per cent sweeter, so you need to eat far less. Refined sugar triggers a surge in insulin, the principal hormone controlling the amount of glucose in the body. But this sudden blood sugar surge tails off rapidly, leaving the body feeling hungry again. Fructose, on the other hand, is absorbed more slowly and produces a steadier and more sustained supply of energy. Studies at Yale University in Connecticut have shown that fruit sugars can also dull the appetite. Clinical trials involving volunteers drinking plain water sweetened with fructose ate significantly less than those who drank either plain water alone or water sweetened with sucrose (refined sugar). It is certainly true that a dose of fructose in the form of an apple eaten twenty minutes before a meal does seem to subdue hunger pangs. On a further health note, clinical studies also show that using fructose in place of refined sugar results in less dental decay and fewer fillings.

Those who avoid eating fresh fruit because they find it difficult to digest may simply be eating it at the wrong time of day. According to Harvey Diamond, the American author of *Fit For Life* (Bantam Books), a best-selling guide to 'food combining', it is important to eat foods in the correct combination. The theory is that fruit takes less energy to be eaten than any other type of food because it is not actually digested in the stomach, but is broken down by the digestive juices before it even gets there. This means that the fruit pulp passes swiftly through the intestines where it can release its nutrients directly into the system. This can only happen, however, if fruit is eaten on an empty stomach, otherwise its passage becomes delayed by the other foods you've eaten which are likely to use a different digestive process. The food combining rules for eating fruit are simple: stick to only fruit before midday as it requires less energy to digest than other foods and is the gentlest way to 'break the fast' at breakfast. At other times of the day only eat fruit on an empty stomach, i.e. just before a meal or four hours afterwards. Harvey Diamond writes with evangelical zeal in his attempt to convert young and old alike to his dietary ideas and claims that fruit is the most beneficial, life-enhancing food there is. He is not alone and there is even a Fruit-arian Society devoted to promoting healthy living by a diet of simple fruits.

Juice Therapy

Fresh fruit juices have been used as a form of therapy for thousands of years and many of mankind's earliest medicines were made from crushed berries and other fruits. Today, technology tells us that the therapeutic elements found in fruit juices are very real and include the powerful antioxidant vitamins e.g. beta carotene, vitamins C and E, and many essential minerals. The revival of treating disease with the use of fresh fruit juices was pioneered in America by Dr Max Gerson, one of the founding 'nature cure' practitioners who successfully cured cancer patients with a raw food diet.

Raw fruit juices are packed with nutrients such as enzymes that are easily destroyed by heat and light, which explains why purists insist on freshly prepared juices that come straight from the fruit, not from the bottle, carton or tin. Also, you may find the contents of packaged juices may not be as pure as they seem. In 1987 an international juice-giant pleaded guilty to over two hundred charges connected with selling an artificially created product which claimed to be 100 per cent pure apple juice. The drink was found to consist of cane sugar, beet sugar, corn syrup, water, and yes, a small amount of apple juice. Since then, the Government has monitored the contents of cartoned juices a little more carefully, but the fact remains that the only way to drink pure, fresh fruit juice is to squeeze your own.

Fresh citrus juices are the easiest of all to obtain by using an electric orange squeezer or simply squeezing them by hand. Other fruit juices can only be extracted by using a centrifugal juice extractor, which is an electric processor that grinds slices of fruit against a whirring sieve to separate the juice from the fibrous part of the plant. These are about the same price as an electric blender and are an excellent investment for any kitchen. The difference between freshly pressed and pre-packaged juices is phenomenal and once you have tasted freshly squeezed apple, pear, mango, melon, pineapple and grape juices you will never want to touch the cartoned stuff again! Juice extractors can also be used to press the juice from many vegetables, including carrots, beetroot, peppers, spinach and celery. Even herbs such as basil and parsley can go through the juicer and you can create the most fabulous fruit and vegetable blends.

Those without juice extractors can still buy many unusual juices pre-squeezed, including apricot, carrot and celery. It is probably better to opt for those sold in glass bottles as there is a possibility that traces of aluminium from the plastic-coated foil used to line some cartons may be absorbed into the juice.

Because juices are a highly concentrated source of nourishment, they should be drunk sparingly. Just as you would not eat 1.5 kg (3 lb) of mango in one go, so you should err on the side of frugality with these fabulous drinks. By all means enjoy them, but don't go overboard or else your digestion might start to rebel. Fresh juices should also be sipped, not slurped in great gulpfuls, and it's better to swirl them around the mouth a little so they mix with digestive enzymes in the saliva before being swallowed.

Juice Cocktails

You can have a lot of fun experimenting with unusual combinations. Here are some deliciously different cocktails to start you off. Stir together equal quantities of the following juices, or adjust the proportions according to personal preference:

Apple and plum
Orange, apple and carrot
Apricot, apple and orange
Pear, apple and mango
Pineapple, apple and kiwi
Orange, carrot and parsley
Apple, tomato and celery
Carrot, watercress and a dash of lemon
Apple, red pepper and a few fresh basil leaves

Apple

That time-honoured expression, 'an apple a day keeps the doctor away', is indeed based on solid fact, and moden medical research can now reveal the attributes of our favourite fruit. Apples originated in the mountains of the Caucases in Russia and have been cultivated in Britain since the Stone Age. The Ancient Egyptians also cultivated apple trees and by the end of the fourth century there were thirty-seven different varieties recorded – today there are well over 1000. For all this, Bramley apples can only be cultivated in Britain, despite efforts to grow them overseas, which explains why apple pie is one of our national dishes.

Apples contain beta carotene and vitamin C as well as small amounts of potassium, calcium and magnesium. They also contain malic and tartaric acid which aids digestion by neutralising the acid by-products of indigestion and helping the body cope with excess protein in rich foods. This is probably why a tart apple sauce is the traditional accompaniment to fatty foods such as roast pork or goose. Apples also contain pectin and several studies have shown that this helps keep our cholesterol levels stable. One French study showed that by eating two apples a day we could expect our cholesterol levels to fall by up to 10 per cent. Research in the United States has also shown that pectin can protect the body from the effects of pollution by binding with heavy metals such as lead and mercury and carrying them safely out of the system. One of Europe's most renowned health practitioners, Dr Bircher-Benner, based his acclaimed wholefood diet cures on the therapeutic properties of apples. He included grated apples in his famous Bircher muesli (see page 168) and used this to treat patients with severe digestive disorders. More recent laboratory experiments using apple juice were carried out by virologist Dr Jack Konowalchuk at Canada's Bureau of Microbial Hazards. He added a wide range of viruses grown in tissue-cell cultures to several different fruit juices, including apple juice. After twenty-four hours, almost all traces of the viruses had disappeared.

Apples are a versatile fruit and can be eaten plain, grated onto cereal or chopped into salads, or they can be lightly cooked to make Apple Crumble (see page 206) or a healthy fruit purée. Eating apples may be used for stewing as well as cooking varieties and because of their natural sweetness these need no added sugar. A favourite form of baby food, apple purée hit the headlines in 1990 when comedienne Pamela Stephenson pioneered the pressure group Parents For Safe Food (PFSF). The woman who has been described as outrageous was herself outraged to learn that the apples and apple juice she had been conscientiously feeding her children contained traces of the powerful pesticide daminozide. With money raised by PFSF, Pamela had raw apples, apple juice and apple sauce from supermarket shelves tested. Worryingly high levels of the pesticide were found in baby foods, amongst other products, and after an intense pressure campaign it was withdrawn from the market – but only after large amounts of the chemical compound had been found to cause cancer in some laboratory animals. Unlike chemical additives which appear on labels in the form of E numbers, we currently have no way of knowing whether our fruit contains traces of toxic pesticides, fertilisers or insecticides. Until such a time when all fruit carries a history of how it was cultivated, by far the safest option is to choose organically grown produce (more about organics on page 112). Shiny apples, although more attractive, may also have been sprayed with a waxy fungicide that gives them a glossy coating and prolongs their shelf life. On balance, it is safer to choose those that do not reveal your reflection. Although pricier than conventional crops, organic apples are less expensive if bought in bulk and late season varieties keep well over the winter if wrapped individually in newspaper and kept in a cool, airy place away from the damp.

Apricot

Fresh apricots are a good source of vitamin C and beta carotene. Apricots have an abundant store of beta carotene which gives them their naturally bright orange colour. As well as being an important vitamin, beta carotene is also the natural pigment that turns produce such as apricots, carrots and mangoes a vivid shade of orange. Beta carotene also combines with the green chlorophyll in many plants to darken their colour, for example, cabbage, courgettes and green beans. As a general rule, the more colourful the produce, the more beta carotene it contains. In addition to their vitamins, fresh apricots are also a rich source of potassium and calcium.

Dried apricots are a useful source of iron and calcium, high in potassium and also contain some beta carotene. However, those that are bright yellow or orange are likely to have been treated with sulphur dioxide which blocks the body's ability to absorb thiamin (vitamin B1) and to which some people such as asthmatics are highly sensitive. It is preferable to buy unsulphured, dried apricots from health food shops, even though they may look less attractive.

Dried Hunza apricots, complete with stones, can also be found in health food shops and before use these need either to be soaked for three to four hours, or simmered for five minutes in just enough water to cover them. Hunza apricots come from Kashmir where they are spread out to dry naturally in the hot sunshine on the corrugated iron roofs of the houses. They have a sweet, nutty flavour and are delicious stewed with a little water and served with a sprinkling of ground almonds. Hunza apricots are often used in Middle Eastern recipes and go well with spicy chick peas and recipes made with pulses and beans. Apricots are also a delicious accompaniment to chicken dishes and are a flavoursome way to extend an otherwise ordinary chicken casserole. Try cracking the stones in Hunza apricots and eating the tasty almond-flavoured kernel. All varieties of apricot kernels contain valuable oil which is extracted industrially by grinding the kernels and siphoning off the oil. This oil is a useful source of both essential fatty acids and vitamin E and may be taken in capsule form. Apricot kernel oil can also be used directly on the skin as a skin soother as it is very easily absorbed.

In addition to their beta carotene supplies, apricots are also a rich source of another group of vitamins called bioflavanoids. These micro-nutrients go hand in hand with vitamin C and the two are always found in foods together.

Banana

Botanically speaking, the banana grows as a herb and not a tree and was one of mankind's first cultivated fruits. Bananas are nature's own form of fast food and are handy to pack in lunch-boxes or take when travelling. Currently our second most popular fruit after apples, bananas are now a national favourite despite only being introduced to Britain just after the Second World War. Naturally high in potassium, bananas also contain reasonable levels of magnesium, phosphorus, beta carotene, folic acid and vitamin C. Bananas have high levels of natural fibre, including pectin which binds with toxins and helps to remove them from the system. The average banana contains only about 95 calories and so slimmers need not worry that bananas are too fattening. Bananas should only be eaten when they are very ripe (wait until their skin begins to turn black) as they are indigestible if the skin is still green. Most bananas imported into Britain arrive bright green and are artificially ripened by gassing, although un-gassed bananas are increasingly available from health food shops and organic produce suppliers. Bananas are a good first food for babies and are as easy to prepare as opening a jar or packet of processed food. Try mixing a mashed banana with a little low-fat, live yoghurt (or soya yoghurt) and a sprinkling of finely ground almonds for a tasty, calcium-enriched children's dessert. Peeled bananas may also be frozen on sticks as additive-free 'ice lollies', or blended with yoghurt and frozen to make a smooth, rich ice-cream.

Blackcurrants

Blackcurrants are one of our richest sources of vitamin C, although raw blackcurrants have over four times as much vitamin C as those canned in syrup or juice. However, all forms of blackcurrants, including those that have been stewed, will pro-vide you with relatively high levels of this valuable nutrient. Blackcurrants also contain useful levels of the minerals potas-sium, calcium and phosphorus. Their black skins are darkened with certain pigments known as anthocynosides, which have anti-bacterial and anti-inflammatory properties, which is why sipping blackcurrant juice mixed with a little hot water is especially sooth-ing for sore throats.

Research published in *Experimental Gerontology* (the study of ageing) in 1982 in Cardiff found that blackcurrant juice signifi-cantly increased the life-span of ageing female mice. This may be due in part to its high vitamin C levels but also to the anthocy-nocides which seem to have a protective effect on blood vessels too. By looking after our blood vessels we not only ward off serious disorders such as heart disease but also maintain our hair and skin with optimum levels of nutrients delivered via the blood supply. Blackcurrants may be stewed with a dash of apple juice to add natural sweetness, or sprinkled raw over salads and desserts for a touch of tang.

Blueberries

Otherwise known as bilberries, whortleberries or huckleberries, blueberries also contain anthocynocides but unlike blackcurrants where they are present only in the outer skin, they occur throughout the entire blueberry fruit. Anthocynocides have the ability to wipe out the *E. coli* bacterium which is a frequent cause of diarrhoea. According to Rodale's *Encyclopaedia of Natural Home Remedies* (Rodale Press), blueberries are a potent cure for diarrhoea. This is confirmed by Professor Finn Sandberg at Uppsala Biomedical Centre in Sweden where blueberries have been used to treat diarrhoea in children. Joint studies between researchers in Paris and Budapest have also established a link between blueberries and low cholesterol levels, possibly because of their pectin content.

Wild blueberries are smaller and tastier than their cultivated companions and both types freeze well. Serve, after rinsing, straight from the punnet or wrapped in Buckwheat Pancakes (see page 166) and a squeeze of fresh lime juice. Blueberries have a longer shelf life than many fruits and may be stored at the top of the fridge for a week or more. They also travel well so they are a good addition to a lunchbox. They are delicious blended into milk or soya milk for a summer milk shake.

Citrus Fruits

Grapefruits the Sri Indians call these *shamees hamt cahaacol* which means 'oranges that enlarge breasts' – a safer but somewhat less effective alternative to silicone. The Roman writer Pliny (the Elder) was the first to use the word 'citrus' to describe grapefruit in his *Historia Naturalis* (written around AD 70) and he classified the fruit as a medicine because of its health-giving properties (now known to be vitamin C). A relatively new citrus fruit, the grapefruit was not officially named until 1830 and almost all of the world's supplies are now grown in America.

Grapefruits contain potassium, calcium, phosphorus, vitamin C and beta carotene, although pink varieties contain sixteen times more beta carotene than the more usual yellow varieties. In addition to their vitamins, grapefruits are also a useful source of the soluble fibre called pectin that can help control cholesterol levels. Studies in America have shown that those who ate 15 g (½ oz) of grapefruit pectin a day in capsules for four months had an average drop of 8 per cent in their total cholesterol levels. Unfortunately, it is not easy to be sure how much pectin is contained within the average grapefruit as it can vary dramatically according to its size, variety and degree of ripeness. However, half a grapefruit eaten for breakfast is likely to do us some good.

Lemons and limes they cured the British navy of life-threatening scurvy, a nutritional disease causing bleeding under the skin as a result of a lack of vitamin C. In 1775, long before vitamin C had been identified, the globe-trotting discoverer Captain James Cook included citrus fruits as part of his crew's sea rations (hence the expression 'limey' which refers to the limes issued to British seamen). Thanks to Captain Cook's foresight, only one of his sailors died, not bad in an age when just half the crew were expected to return to shore alive.

In addition to their vitamin C levels, lemons and limes also contain bioflavanoids in their skins and pulp. The only snag is that the skin of most fruits is also coated with a wax containing a fungicide which gives them an unnaturally glossy shine and lengthens their shelf life. So bear this in mind when using slices, or the peel. In Germany, lemons, limes and oranges that have been sprayed carry a warning not to use their peel, but British labelling standards are less vigilant. Buy un-waxed fruits whenever possible or scrub them well with diluted washing-up liquid before use to remove as much of the waxy coating as possible. Alternatively, buy organically grown citrus fruit.

Oranges These are one of our most common sources of vitamin C and both fresh oranges and freshly squeezed orange juice contain high levels of this valuable nutrient. In studies carried out by the National Cancer Institute in America those who ate the most oranges, compared to those who ate the fewest, had the lowest incidence of developing cancer. Vitamin C seems to have an important role to play in fighting cancer as it inhibits powerful carcinogens known as nitrosamines that crop up in some foods, notably bacon and pork products. Vitamin C is also a major component of collagen, the protein fibres that support the skin. As an antioxidant nutrient, it also helps to neutralise the free radicals that contribute to the visible signs of premature ageing such as skin sagging and wrinkles. In Florida, where much of America's crop is grown, researchers have noted that orange pith is also one of our most accessible sources of pectin. Orange pith is also rich in bioflavanoids.

Orange juice is best drunk freshly squeezed from the fruit as it oxidises with the air and quickly turns acidic. Not only is cartoned orange juice more acidic, but even those labelled 'pure orange juice' may contain a few surprises. A 1991 survey by the Ministry of Agriculture found that several well-known brands of cartoned 'juice' contained added sugar, malic acid and pulpwash (made by soaking the left-over orange skins in water and giving them another good squeeze to make orange-flavoured water). Unfortunately, levels of fungicides were not tested at the time but given that virtually all oranges are sprayed before harvesting it can be assumed that some traces would also be present in the final product.

Fresh orange juice not only supplies the body with vitamin C but also increases iron absorption by up to three times. Drinking a glass of orange juice with your breakfast cereal or boiled egg actually doubles the amount of iron available in the bloodstream. To avoid waste, small amounts of left-over orange or lemon juice can be poured into ice-cube trays and frozen for future use.

Cherries

The cherry tree is closely related to the plum and peach and its fruits may be sweet or sour depending on the species. The Ancient Greeks prescribed cherries for epilepsy, gallstones and gout, and while there is no medical evidence to support their theories we do know that cherries are a good source of the powerful antioxidant, vitamin C. Raw cherries contain ten times as much vitamin C as those canned in syrup and the new cherry orchards in Kent will make British cherries more easily available – and cheaper than imported fruits. Cherries should always be thoroughly washed to remove any traces of insecticide sprays. They freeze well so take advantage of the glut that comes on to the market during the summer and stock up for the year ahead.

Cranberries

As well as the fresh form, dried cranberries are also becoming more widely available, and these are significantly sweeter than fresh crops as their fructose content is more highly concentrated.

Cranberries are high in beta carotene and vitamin C as well as containing iron, potassium and unique bacteria-fighting substances that can help treat urinary tract infections, including painful cystitis. At first this was thought to be due to the cranberries increasing the amount of hippuric acid in the urine which kills off bacterium. However, researchers at Youngstown State University, Ohio, have found that, in fact, cranberries and cranberry juice seems to prevent *E. coli*, the rogue organism responsible for most urinary infections and diarrhoea, from sticking to the cells in the bladder and the urethra by wrapping them in a kind of non-stick coating. Dr Anthony Sobota, a microbiology professor at the Youngstown State University, has also reported that cranberries have an antibiotic action within the body. It's not surprising, therefore, that some naturopaths now treat urinary disorders with cranberry juice, thus avoiding conventional antibiotics. Research carried out by the leading cranberry producers has revealed that just one small glass of cranberry juice a day can ward off urinary tract and bladder infections in those who are prone to them.

Dates

Bedouin tribes travelled for days across the desert with little more than a handful of dates to keep them going. Naturally sweet, fresh dates are highly nutritious and make a tasty lunchbox snack. Both fresh and dried dates are high in fibre and help to remove impurities from the system by countering constipation. Dried dates may also be purchased pressed into a block which is useful for slicing into salads or chopping off small amounts for other recipes. Look out for the unsulphured varieties if you can.

Figs

The Romans were fond of feasting on figs, although the best fruits were kept for the emperors who favoured their rich, purple flesh (purple was the colour reserved exclusively for the imperial family). The Roman historian Pliny was also fond of the fig and wrote, 'figs are restorative and the best food that can be taken by those who are brought low by long sickness'. According to Jean Harper, author of *The Food Pharmacy* (Simon and Schuster), modern medics are now looking more closely into the medicinal properties of this unusual fruit. She cites Japanese scientists at the Institute of Physical and Chemical Research at the Mitsubishi-Kasei Institute of Life Sciences in Tokyo, who have isolated an anti-cancer chemical from figs. Fifty-five patients with advanced cancer improved when injected with this substance, called benzaldehyde, with seven patients going into total remission and twenty-nine into partial remission. Other experiments using plain fig juice reveal that it can kill bacterium when drunk or even applied externally.

Fig trees can survive for several centuries and are a common sight in the Mediterranean and the tropics. Fresh figs are imported year-round into Britain, although they are at their cheapest in the autumn. Fresh figs contain beta carotene and vitamin C as well as traces of calcium and zinc. Dried figs have more concentrated levels of potassium (essential for skin cells) and calcium (important for bone maintenance), although most are dried using sulphur dioxide and many also have sugar added. Both fresh and dried figs contain the enzyme *ficin*, that aids digestion, have plenty of natural fibre and are a mild laxative.

Grapefruit (see **Citrus fruits** page 94).

Grapes

Grapes are mostly water with traces of vitamins and minerals, notably potassium, which make them excellent internal cleansers. One-day grape fasts occasionally are a useful way to de-toxify the system and the South African naturopath Johanna Brandt, author of *The Grape Cure* (now out of print), claims to have cured herself of cancer by eating nothing but grapes for several months. Fasting clinics in Germany including Dr Buchinger's centre in Bad Pyrmont and Dr Heide's clinic in Laasphe frequently use grapes as a simple seven-day, supervised single-fruit fast and report good results for patients with arthritis as well as the more obvious benefits of substantial weight loss.

Since the introduction of seedless grapes our consumption has soared to an average per person of 2.25 kg (5 lb) per year. The newest varieties to hit the shelves include larger black, white, and red varieties and juicy muscat-flavoured grapes. However, as most grapes are frequently sprayed during cultivation it is important either to wash them thoroughly or to choose organically produced varieties. The United Farm Workers of America have frequently called for a boycott of Californian grapes to put pressure on those grape growers who insist on using pesticides known to be toxic both to the grape pickers who harvest the crops and to the consumer who eats them.

Kiwi

Known as the Chinese gooseberry until the New Zealanders hijacked it in the seventies and exported the 'kiwi' to nouvelle cuisine restaurants round the world. The new generation of kiwi fruit is now grown in Italy and France and these varieties have a slightly sweeter flavour than the original antipodean version which can still sometimes be found in supermarkets. The New Zealanders are currently experimenting with hybrid varieties and in the future we can expect to see fuzz-free kiwi and even pastel pink ones. Hopefully these perversions of nature will not impair its nutritional value as despite its slightly shabby fur coat, the average kiwi contains more vitamin C than an orange. Kiwi fruits are also a useful source of beta carotene and many minerals including potassium, calcium and phosphorus. Its gorgeous green colour is a favourite with gourmets and while it brightens up fruit salads and flans, slices of kiwi fruit also work well in savoury salads. Children also enjoy kiwis served whole like a boiled egg – simply slice the top off and scoop out the insides.

Lemons and limes (see **Citrus fruits** page 94).

Mango

The magnificent mango contains high levels of beta carotene with useful amounts of vitamin C and potassium, and its greeny-red skin has become a familiar sight in the supermarket over recent years. Mangoes have proved to be a hit with the British public and we now eat well over fifty million a year. With huge new plantations in South America and Israel coming into production, the Fresh Fruit and Vegetable Association is confidently predicting a mango boom. When choosing a mango, reject any that are bruised or damaged and sniff for the unmistakably sweet scent that indicates it is ripe. Once picked though, the mango ripens slowly and you may need to wait patiently for weeks rather than days for it to become soft and juicy.

The neatest way to chop a mango into bite-sized chunks for fruit salad is to cut it in half across the middle, each side of the stone (cutting the rounded ends off), turn each portion 'inside-out' and cut a crisscross pattern deep into the flesh. Slice the cubes into a bowl. Diced mango is a good substitute for summer's soft fruits and gives an exotic touch to plain yoghurt, muesli or pancakes. Its naturally sweet flavour goes down well with children and chunks of mango can also be used to make a fast, raw fruit purée. Slices of fresh mango work well with savoury dishes and are delicious served with chicken or ham.

Melon

Melons are now available all year round and are imported from France, Spain and Israel. Several varieties are commonly available, including the honeydew melon which has a tough yellow casing and is shaped like a rugby ball; the galia melon which is smaller and is surrounded by a buff-coloured webbing; the cantaloupe melons, including the charentais, which are also small and orange-fleshed; and the ogen melon, named after the kibbutz where it was developed and which has a yellow skin and a pale green inside. Their nutritional values vary according to type as each variety contains different quantities of nutrients. For example, the peach-coloured flesh of the canteloupe has twenty times as much beta carotene and three times as much vitamin C as the paler honeydew. Epidemiological studies that compare diet against incidence of cancer consistently show that those who eat plenty of fresh green and yellow fruits (such as melons) are less likely to die from cancer, and beta carotene is widely believed to be the key. In addition to its vitamin content, cantaloupe melon is also a reasonable source of potassium and calcium.

As melon quickly ferments in the stomach unless it can pass unimpeded through the digestive system it is best either to eat melon just on its own or with only another soft fruit, or at the beginning of a meal. Melon is the simplest fruit to serve and half a melon with the seeds scooped out and filled with strawberries makes a quick and attractive starter. A melon cocktail made by marinating chunks of melon in freshly squeezed orange juice and grated, fresh ginger root will also wake up the taste-buds and get the digestive juices flowing. You could even invest in a melon-baller, a nifty gadget that carves perfect spheres for superior serving ideas. Try arranging multi-coloured melon balls carved from several different varieties and garnishing them with a sprig of mint. Or how about a refreshing melon jelly with this idea adapted from a recipe by vegetarian cookery writer, Rose Elliott: place a few melon balls in a glass bowl, bring (600 ml) 1 pint apple or white or red grape juice to the boil, remove from the heat and sprinkle in 2 teaspoons of agar agar (a seaweed gelling agent). Whisk until dissolved, then bring back to the boil for one minute. Allow to cool slightly before pouring over the melon balls and leave to set.

Papaya

Also known as the paw paw, the salmon-pink flesh of this fruit has a tender texture and melt-in-the-mouth consistency, similar to the avocado. Inside, the papaya houses a multitude of dark, shiny pips which have a slightly peppery flavour. Papaya contains high levels of beta carotene (hence its orangey-pink colour), significant amounts of vitamin C, potassium and some calcium. This tropical delicacy also contains the enzyme papain, which helps digest protein. Slices of papaya can be used in a marinade to tenderise tougher cuts of meat. Or try wrapping chicken breasts or lamb chops in papaya skins and leaving them overnight in the fridge. The next day brush the meat with a mixture of olive oil and freshly crushed garlic or grated, fresh ginger root and cook it under the grill.

Papaya is at its best when it's soft and very ripe. Its flavour works well when contrasted with the sharpness of citrus fruits. Serve slices of papaya with a wedge of lemon or lime to squeeze over, or mix chunks of papaya with orange and grapefruit segments for a refreshing fresh fruit compote.

Passion Fruit

Despite its sexy name, passion fruit is known more for spirituality than sensuality as it was christened by Catholic priests to illustrate the crucifixion or 'passion' of Christ. The deep purple flowers have a group of central filaments that resemble the crown of thorns, while the stigma is in the shape of the cross with the stamens representing the nails. The passion fruit plant is native to South America and was later cultivated in the Mediterranean. It needs a sunny, south-facing wall to grow in Britain and you are unlikely to get any fruit unless it is grown under glass. The leaves and flowering tops of the plant have been used by herbalists for centuries and have powerful anti-spasmodic and relaxant properties. Passiflora extract is a herbal narcotic with a similar chemical composition to morphine. It is often combined with other calming herbs such as scullcap and valerian to make a powerful sedating brew. In Romania a patent has been granted for a sedative chewing gum that contains passiflora extract.

Although the passion fruits themselves do not have the same effect as the leaves and flowers on our physique they do contain valuable nutrients, including B vitamins, beta carotene, vitamin C, potassium and phosphorus. Unlike our own complexion, the more wrinkles on the skin of these small brown fruits the better. Their deceptively frugal insides consist of little more than a small spoonful of slippery yellow pips in a scented, cerise substance. Once you have tasted fresh, ripe passion fruit juice (made simply by sieving the contents) no other sauce will ever so successfully top your Buckwheat Pancakes (see page 166) or fresh fruit sorbet. Passion fruit juice is also delicious when it's mixed with freshly squeezed orange juice and a splash of sparkling mineral water for a subtly scented, fizzy fruit cocktail.

The pips in passionfruit are also processed industrially and a skin-care oil is extracted. Taking passionflower oil (bought in capsule form) is an excellent way to promote skin elasticity as it contains a high percentage of linoleic acid, the essential fatty acid that literally holds the skin together.

Peach

Peaches were first cultivated over four thousand years ago and are thought to have originated in China. They were called 'Persian plums' by the Romans who used poultices of ground peach kernels to drive out worms! The peach tree likes a limey soil with plenty of strong sunshine in the summer months, and cold, dry winters. If the climatic conditions are right, the peach tree can happily thrive for several hundred years. Peaches need many hours of sunshine to ripen and are ready for harvesting towards the end of the summer. The fruits are then exported whole, or sliced open prior to the canning process which leaves the kernels available for their oil to be extracted. Peach kernel oil is a light golden oil containing useful amounts of essential fatty acids and vitamin E. It is used as a base ingredient in many moisturisers and aromatherapy massage blends and is an excellent skin softener. Peaches have only been available in Britain during this century and the first consignment to arrive at Covent Garden market was from Ontario, Canada in 1909. Peaches are an excellent source of the antioxidant beta carotene and also contain useful amounts of the minerals potassium and phosphorus. Peaches can easily be used in recipes instead of apricots, or are delicious eaten just as they are. Those who object to their fuzzy skins can easily blanch the fruit first for a few seconds in boiling water before running it under the cold tap and peeling it.

Pear

Another British staple, the pear contains useful amounts of beta carotene, vitamin C and potassium. Delicious raw or stewed, several different varieties are now widely available. The sweeter dessert pears include the yellow-skinned William's pear and the slightly rounder comice pear. The conference pear is also a popular British variety recognised by its tougher greenish-brown skin. This type is useful for cooking and stewed pears or pear purée can both be frozen. Pear sauce, made simply by cooking and sieving the fruit, works surprisingly well with many vegetarian dishes, including veggie burgers, nut rissoles and savoury lentil dishes. Raw pears can be chopped into salads or grated into plain yoghurt for a fresh, fruity, dessert that goes down well with babies and children. Those fortunate enough to have a centrifugal fruit juicer are also likely to develop a healthy addiction to freshly pressed pear juice.

Pineapple

This tropical delicacy is really a cluster of tiny fruits that bond together as they grow. Raw pineapple contains many nutrients, notably beta carotene, folic acid, vitamin C, potassium, calcium and magnesium. Fresh pineapple also contains the enzyme bromalin which counteracts bacterium and helps to keep the gut free from infection. Bromalin also helps with the digestion of protein which explains why a small amount of pineapple eaten at the end of a meal can improve the digestion of protein-rich foods. However, it's the same enzyme that inhibits the use of pineapple in jellies as it dissolves the gelatine proteins and prevents setting. Bromalin is such a powerful enzyme that workers in canning factories have to wear protective gloves to stop their skin from being eaten away by the juice. However, once it's within the digestive tract, bromalin only acts on food and dead tissues, leaving our insides in good order.

The clues to look for when choosing a fresh pineapple are a sweet, fruity smell and leaves that can be easily pulled away from the crown. Fresh pineapple chunks are good served with freshly squeezed orange juice. Decorate with mint leaves for a refreshing taste bud treat. Although tinned pineapple loses its bromalin content in the canning process, it still retains some of its nutrients but I suggest that if you are buying tinned chunks, you look for those packed in natural fruit juice instead of sugar syrup.

Plums And Prunes

Rich in beta carotene, potassium and phosphorus with some vitamin C, plums are a nutritious food. Raw plums contain just over ten times as much beta carotene and four times as much vitamin C as those canned in syrup.

Ready-to-eat prunes, made from a variety of black-skinned plums, also contain more vitamins and minerals than tinned varieties and are a useful source of beta carotene, calcium and iron. Watch out for prunes that appear unnaturally shiny though, as these may have been coated with mineral oil to improve their appearance. Although this additive prevents the prunes from sticking together it also inhibits the absorption of minerals when you eat them. The answer is either to scrub off the mineral oil or to buy other brands. Infamous for their laxative effect, this is due to the prune's peculiar chemical composition which explains why drinking prune juice (which no longer contains any fibre) also acts as a laxative in the system. There is little doubt that adding prunes or prune juice to the diet is a more natural and nutritious option for those who otherwise depend on artificial laxatives. The chief complaint with prunes, however, is wind and stomach cramps and the best way round this is to eat prunes sparingly at first, allowing the system time to adjust to their powerful effect before eating more than a couple at a time. The discomfort usually passes after two to three weeks, so if constipation is a severe problem it is worth persevering with the prunes! However, those who tend towards constipation will find that their digestive system improves while following the suggestions in this book because of the emphasis on high-fibre and water-filled foods.

Rhubarb

Technically an edible stem and not a fruit, rhubarb is a nutritious food and time-honoured internal cleanser and natural tonic. Even rhubarb that has been stewed at moderate temperatures contains reasonable amounts of beta carotene, folic acid and vitamin C. It is also surprisingly high in calcium but because rhubarb is also high in oxalic acid (which combines with calcium to form insoluble calcium oxalate) this calcium is not absorbed by the body. Rhubarb should be prepared by discarding the leaves (which contain concentrated oxalic acid and are poisonous) and trimming away any tough pieces of stalk. It can then be simmered in a little water and flavoured with cinnamon sticks, grated, fresh ginger root, or freshly squeezed orange juice, adding date syrup (available in a bottle from health food shops) as the sweetener. You can also boost the nutritional value of other fruit juices by mixing them with the leftover cooking liquid.

Soft Fruits

Blackberries one of the first fruits eaten by man, blackberries were mentioned by the Ancient Greek 'father of medicine' Hippocrates mentioned their use as both a food and a medicine as long ago as 400 BC. Blackberries are a good source of vitamin C but beware of picking those that grow on the roadside as the fruits absorb the poisonous carbon monoxide from car exhausts. All soft fruits, including blackberries, should be gently washed by placing them in a sieve and rolling them in a basin of water to dislodge dirt and dust without causing damage. They can then be dried on sheets of kitchen paper. Blackberries are marvellous mixed with apple purée or in Apple Crumble (see page 206) or made into a delicious, dark coulis to go with poached pears or fruit salad by simmering them until soft, then passing them through a sieve. Personally, I make sure I use blackberries which are ripe and sweet enough, without adding sugar or any other sweetener. Blackberry juice can also be added to fresh fruit cocktails for an unusually rich flavour.

Raspberries an excellent source of vitamin C, raspberries also contain useful amounts of potassium and calcium. According to leading practitioner of alternative medicine Michael van Straten, raspberries should be on every hospital menu as they not only supply useful nutrients but are also particularly easy to digest. Raspberries can be prepared and eaten the same way as blackberries but are also hard to beat simply eaten as they are.

Strawberries a good source of vitamin C, beta carotene, potassium, calcium and iodine, these ruby red jewels also contain useful amounts of the plant fibre pectin. As with most fruits, studies suggest that those eating a diet high in strawberries are less likely to develop cancer. They have also been linked to relieving arthritis and the renowned Swedish botanist, Linnaeus, fasted on strawberries alone to cure his own arthritis successfully. He attributed their healing powers to an unusually purifying and cleansing action within the system. As with melons, strawberries break down very quickly in the stomach and should ideally be eaten either alone or only with other soft fruits, or at the very beginning of a meal. British strawberries are only available for six to eight weeks a year, although supplies are flown in year-round from Israel and California. Because of their short shelf life, strawberries were some of the first fruits to be irradiated, although any that have been zapped should be clearly marked and avoided because of their lack of vitamins and potential free radical problems. Fresh strawberries need little preparation (see blackberries for washing) and are the perfect fruit to slice into salads of all descriptions. They can also be stewed with a little water, ground almonds and a drop or two of natural almond essence for a nutritious dessert. Strawberries freeze well if they are spread out on a baking sheet and the frozen fruits make great 'ice-cubes' for fresh fruit cocktails.

Fresh Fruit Fact Finder

Fresh fruits are nature's own vitamin pills as they contain high levels of vitamin C together with several other nutrients. The orange and yellow fruits such as cantaloupe melons, apricots and papaya are rich in the anti-oxidant beta carotene, and all fruits are naturally low in sodium (salt) and have good levels of potassium. This is important for maintaining the body's potassium-to-sodium ratio which is often out of balance due to our high intake of salty foods.

Fruit is also an excellent source of dietary fibre, including soluble fibre that helps control cholesterol levels in the bloodstream. Dietary fibre is also useful for preventing constipation and helps keep our internal organs functioning healthily.

Fruit	Fibre Content*	Vitamin C Content*	Additional Nutrients*
Apple (each)	2 g	4 mg	
Apricot (each)	3 g	7 mg	beta carotene
Bananas (each)	4 g	11 mg	iron, the B vitamins pyridoxine and folic acid
Blackberry*	8 g	22 mg	rich in calcium, magnesium and iron
Blackcurrant	8.5 g	188 mg	vitamin E, rich in calcium and magnesium
Blueberry	2.5 g	16 mg	iron
Cantaloupe Melon	1 g	30 mg	rich in beta carotene
Cherry	1.5 g	18 mg	iron
Cranberry	4.5 g	12 mg	rich in iron
Date (fresh)	8.5 g	trace	rich in B vitamins, including folic acid, iron
Fig (fresh)	2.5 g	2 mg	good source of calcium
Grape	3 g	5 mg	

Fruit	Fibre Content*	Vitamin C Content*	Additional Nutrients*
Grapefruit	2.5 g	36 mg	
Kiwi	3.5 g	72 mg	iron
Lemon	1.5 g	24 mg	
Mango	2 g	36 mg	iron, rich in beta carotene
Orange	3 g	70 mg	B vitamins thiamin and folic acid. Iron
Passionfruit	4 g	5 mg	
Papaya	2 g	60 mg	iron, rich in beta carotene
Peach	2 g	8 mg	rich in beta carotene
Pear	4 g	5 mg	folic acid
Pineapple	2 g	17 mg	
Plum	2 g	3 mg	vitamin E
Raspberry	8 g	23 mg	rich in iron and magnesium
Rhubarb	2.5 g	8 mg	iron, rich in calcium
Strawberry	2 g	58 mg	folic acid and iron

* per 100 g unless otherwise stated

Sources: *The Encyclopedia of Food and Nutrition* (Merehurst) and *The Composition of Foods* (MAFF)

VITALITY VEGETABLES

Eat yourself beautiful with three varieties each day (in addition to potatoes). Vegetables contain the nutrients that ensure our vim and vigour. From dark leafy greens to the mighty roots and tubers, all vegetables are rich in the fibre that cleanses our system. Vegetables are the mainstay of any healthy eating regime, which is why this plan insists on three different types a day. This is in addition to potatoes, which nutritionists group with other starches such as bread and pasta. Historically, Britons have relied on beans, peas, root vegetables, onions and cabbage as staples to our diet. All other vegetables, such as corn, tomatoes, potatoes and avocados came via the New World countries of America and the Far East. Although vegetables have been eaten for thousands of years, it was not until the discovery of vitamins at the beginning of this century that we realised just how important they are for better health. The most significant vitamins in vegetables are vitamin C and beta carotene (some of which is converted into vitamin A in the body while the rest is used as an antioxidant).

It is becoming clear that vegetables also contain as yet unidentified substances that protect us from cancer. Population studies in the United States show that cancer risks greatly decrease when broccoli, cabbage, carrots, celery, cucumbers, green peppers and tomatoes are added to the diet. Unfortunately, we British are not that keen on eating up our greens and eat less than half the amount consumed by the Spanish and Greeks. This higher vegetable consumption is part of the so-called Mediterranean diet effect, thought to be responsible for the lower rates of heart disease and cancer on the Continent. There is no doubt that fresh vegetables, prepared with the minimum of processing to retain the highest nutrient levels, are a fundamental part of better health and glowing good looks. There is also no question that to get the most from them they should also be organically grown.

Why go organic?

There are many good reasons for choosing organically grown vegetables, fruits and other produce:

> *Organically grown crops contain many more vitamins and minerals.*
>
> *Organic produce does not contain traces of harmful chemical pesticides.*
>
> *Organic farming is good for the environment and therefore benefits our planet.*
>
> *Organically grown produce tastes better!*

It is an undisputed fact of farming life that modern methods of cultivation have grossly contaminated our soil, crops and water supplies with pesticides and chemical fertilisers. These chemicals work by supplying the soil with the basic ingredients for plant growth; nitrogen (in the form of nitrates), phosphorus, potassium and calcium. Unfortunately, by overloading the earth with these elements they disrupt the delicate balance of other vitally important trace elements, such as magnesium and boron. This means that the crops grown in them contain fewer potentially life-saving nutrients (boron, for example, is a bone-strengthening mineral that can help osteoporosis and arthritis). In addition, the excess nitrogen in the soil ends up contaminating our water supplies in the form of cancer-causing nitrates. By contrast, organic farmers use only environmentally friendly fertilisers that include manure, seaweed, herbs such as comfrey and mineral-enriched rock dust to feed the soil with a complete spectrum of nutrients. Crops grown the organic way end up with a higher nutritional content and contain extra protein, more vitamin C and minerals such as calcium and iron. They are also free from chemical pesticides and are not sprayed with toxic fungicides.

Organic Extras

Why take vitamin and mineral pills when organic produce gives you all these extra nutrients?

Iron	+ 290%
Calcium	+ 56%
Magnesium	+ 49%
Essential amino acids	+ 35%
Manganese	+ 28%
Protein	+ 12%
Nitrates	− 69%

Source: *Biological Husbandry* (Butterworths)

The Pesticide Problem

Apart from being nutritionally inferior, conventional crops are also contaminated with pesticides and other chemicals. Pesticides are, by definition, highly toxic to animal life. They also interfere with our absorption of vitamins and minerals from food. Pesticides and other 'aggro-chemicals' such as herbicides and fungicides sprayed on crops fall into two groups. The first are the systemic sprays that enter through the leaves and are distributed evenly throughout the plant. The other group, known as contact-active agents, remain on the plant's surface. Chemicals applied after harvesting, such as mould inhibitors, are likely to remain on the surface, whereas those sprayed on the crops while they are growing are more likely to spread throughout the plant. Most contact-active chemicals can be washed off with soapy water or lost in the peel (although many nutrients will also be removed). However, systemic agents can *never* be washed away and the only way to avoid eating them is to buy organically grown produce.

MORE BAD NEWS

Unlike other chemical additives used during food processing, the pesticide content of a food does not appear on the label. So just how prevalent is the problem? One survey carried out by Parents for Safe Food and Friends of the Earth, in 1990 found high pesticide residues in such basic products as brown bread, crisps and tomato ketchup. When the Association for Public Health Analysts tested 305 different fruits in 1989, more than a third were found to be contaminated with pesticides, some with as many as six different types. In 1992, Government monitoring by the Ministry of Agriculture, Food and Fisheries (MAFF) discovered that one-third of all British carrots contained the pesticide triazophos at levels higher than the Maximum Residue Level (MRL). So how have they tackled this problem? Well, they actually propose to increase the MRL to a level 50 times greater than the World

Health Organisation guidelines. So much for the considerations of the consumer. Another survey reported in *Nutrition and Health* in 1987 found that many other vegetables on sale in the UK exceed the legal limits for pesticides set by other countries.

As many of our vegetables are imported it is worth taking a look at the findings from other countries. Tests in Germany have found that the fungicide vinclozin can cause birth defects and other reproductive problems, yet this chemical is still regularly sprayed on apples, tomatoes, lettuce and peppers. Measurements taken at Italy's largest fruit and vegetable markets have also revealed alarming levels of residues, with almost half the oranges on sale containing large amounts of pesticides. Overall, produce from Spain and Argentina had the highest levels of toxic chemicals. The commonest residues were the pesticides listed as suspected cancer-causing agents by the US Environment Protection Agency and included captan, folpet and benomil.

The insecticide lindane is still widely used in cocoa production in West Africa and residues have cropped up in British manufactured chocolates. An investigation by The *Sunday Mirror* newspaper in 1990 revealed lindane residues in a number of chocolates produced by Britain's leading manufacturers. Although lindane is more of a hazard to those harvesting the cocoa beans than those eating the final product, the chemical is known to build up both in the environment and in the human body. While the traces of lindane found in some chocolates are unlikely to be harmful, they are undesirable. Of course, those following the eating plan in this book probably won't be eating much chocolate, but those who do will be relieved to hear that organic chocolate is now available!

The plight of the cocoa harvesters uncovers another disturbing problem: a review by the Pesticide Health Effects Study Group reported in the medical journal *The Lancet* estimates that around the world, there are 3 million severe cases of pesticide poisoning and 230 000 deaths annually. These occur mainly in underdeveloped countries where economic pressures encourage the ever increasing use of chemicals. And as we import greater amounts of produce from these developing nations, this problem is ultimately served up on our own plates.

THE SAFE OPTION

Pressure groups are one way of focusing Government attention on the domestic and worldwide problem of pesticides. One of the largest is called SAFE, which stands for Sustainable Agriculture, Food and Environment. Launched in 1991, SAFE has the financial backing of businessman Sir James Goldsmith, whose reputation in the corporate food industry has been replaced with that of a greener consciousness. The idea behind SAFE is that organics is a wide issue that includes farming, animal welfare and environmental issues. The organisation supports the theory that farmers should be paid according to how their crops are grown, not by how much is produced. As Hugh Raven, SAFE's co-ordinator says, 'What is so efficient about intensive farming that produces unwanted surpluses and so pollutes our water with pesticides that we (the tax-payer) have to spend hundreds of millions of pounds to clean it up?' What we spend on organic produce now, we save on taxes to clean our water supply later. SAFE claims that agriculture and food policy are at a crossroads and that one way continues to head towards environmental damage and surpluses of unhealthy food. The other route, encompassed in the aims of SAFE, is to produce affordable food, of higher nutritional quality, with the minimum of chemical contaminants. These aims are supported at the highest level by HRH The Prince of Wales, whose own farm at Highgrove in Gloucestershire is run organically.

More generally, a 1988 survey by the National Consumer Council found that 80 per cent of the population might be willing to pay more for crops produced with fewer fertilisers, weedkillers and pesticides. While organic produce does cost more now, the laws of supply and demand dictate that if the demand increases, the prices will come down. Another excellent organisation is The Soil Association, who not only supply information about organic farming to schools and other members of the public, but can also advise on your nearest stockist of organic produce. If you want to find out more about either SAFE or The Soil Association, you will find addresses for more information on page 213.

THE TASTE TEST

Not only are organically grown vegetables more nutritious and better for the environment – they taste better too! Although they may sometimes be a slightly odd shape or a duller colour than those covered in chemicals, they undoubtedly have a superior flavour. In a blind tasting session carried out by The *Independent* newspaper in 1992, organic produce won hands down against conventional crops. Amongst the panel of foodies was top chef Nico Ladenis, whose restaurant has received two rare Michelin stars for excellence. The panel tasted winter carrots, boiled white potatoes, comice pears, raw cox's apples, pizza base, fruit cake and organically reared roast chicken. The clearest differences were noted with the vegetables. 'Stunning – I couldn't believe the difference,' said Nico Ladenis on the merits of the organic carrot. The same held true of the organic pears. The organic variety were 'sweet and aromatic' compared to the conventional pear which was deemed to be 'tasteless and grainy'. Overall, those who have tried organic crops, especially vegetables, have found that they really do have a good, old-fashioned flavour.

Raw Versus Cooked

The fastest way to lose the flavour of any vegetable is to overcook it. Not only are over-cooked vegetables soggy and tasteless, they also contain fewer important nutrients. Although vegetables are an excellent source of fibre, carbohydrates and minerals with a handful of vitamins and enzymes thrown in for good measure, the only way to ensure you receive **all** these nutrients is to eat them raw, such as in salads or chopped into sticks for crudités and served with a yoghurt dip. Even gentle heating robs vegetables of their delicate enzymes and some vitamin C. Vitamins are especially vulnerable as they tend to be water soluble and are absorbed into the cooking water during blanching or boiling. Cooking vegetables in a lot of water means that many of their nutrients end up disappearing down the sink. Other nutrients, such as beta carotene and the B vitamins, are also destroyed by heat and may not survive the cooking process. The best way to cook vegetables quickly is to steam them lightly in a steamer over a saucepan containing a little water, or to put them in a covered container in the microwave oven. Vegetables such as carrots and parsnips should be eaten with their skins on as the highest concentration of vitamins and minerals lies just beneath the surface. A stiff scrubbing brush is all that is needed to clean most vegetables and preserve their nutritional content.

Freezing And Canning

All vegetables are at their best when fresh and this is when their nutritional values are at their highest. Whether frozen or canned, all vegetables are first blanched in boiling water to clean them and kill off any bugs. This also knocks out some of their vitamin C levels and kills enzymes. Freezing a vegetable can also damage its cell walls and result in further vitamin loss. Canning is even more damaging as the vegetables are heated and up to 90 per cent of the vitamins A and E may be destroyed. Minerals are more resilient, but around half the magnesium and zinc will be lost if the canning liquid is thrown away. However, lengthy storage times also reduce the vitamin content of fresh produce. Vegetables stored for many months before reaching the shops can contain fewer vitamins than those that have been frozen. For example, frozen peas may well contain more vitamin C than fresh peas that have been badly handled or stored. If vegetables look wilted or you have left the broccoli in the bottom of the fridge for a week then you are probably better off with frozen. The guide is to buy fresh produce when possible and reject any that looks past its best. Fresh vegetables should be eaten within a few days. Don't peel or slice anything until you are ready to cook or eat it. Keep vegetables cool and store salad vegetables in the fridge.

Cabbages And Kings

Many of our most important vegetables belong to the *brassicas* or *cruciferous* group, whose family members include cabbage, Brussels sprouts, broccoli and cauliflower. The most potent of the brassicas is mustard, which contains powerful natural oils. All brassicas are rich in vitamins, minerals and sulphur compounds that benefit the hair and skin.

Cabbage and Brussels sprouts these are a favourite with naturopaths and cabbage juice is often served as a tonic. Raw cabbage juice has also been found to help stomach ulcers and so its mystery ingredient has been codenamed vitamin U. Vitamin-enriched cabbage is easy to find as the darker the leaves, the more beta carotene it contains. In fact, the darker outer leaves can hold up to 30 times as many vitamins than the paler inner leaves, so don't discard them. From both a nutrient point of view and that of preventing that overbearing smell which we associate with overcooked 'greens' you need to cook them quickly in an inch or so of water, or steam them, and serve at once. Lightly boiled cabbage is delicious simmered with a handful of fennel or dill seeds and a teaspoon of olive oil. Brussels sprouts can also be served with chopped dill or fresh coriander leaves and a scattering of cooked chestnuts.

Broccoli and cauliflower these are large stems covered in edible flowers (broccoli) and underdeveloped buds (cauliflower). Broccoli was introduced to the world by Catherine de Medici from Italy. When she set off from Florence in 1533 to marry the heir to the French throne, she took Italian chefs and several varieties of vegetables with her. Amongst these were savoy cabbages, artichokes and broccoli. By 1700 these had been cultivated in Britain and have remained popular ever since.

The Americans are less keen on broccoli and in 1991 President George Bush even banned it from the White House. This caused such a national furore that he was forced to apologise to the

119

broccoli growers. The President is also known to dislike carrots and refers to them in private as 'orange broccoli'.

Broccoli itself is a nutritional giant. It is high in beta carotene and vitamin C, and contains useful amounts of calcium. Scientists from the Johns Hopkins University School of Medicine in Baltimore have also isolated an additional substance that encourages the body to produce the protective enzymes that fight tumours. Dr Paul Talalay says, 'we are very excited about this - and we don't excite easily'. It is hoped that the substance, called sulforaphane, can be concentrated and used to treat those in high-risk cancer groups. Cauliflower and other brassicas also contain this cancer-fighting compound. Cauliflower is a good source of vitamin C but has few other nutrients. Both broccoli and cauliflower are best eaten raw in salads or with a yoghurt dip. Otherwise, they should be lightly steamed and served hot or cold with a squeeze of fresh lemon juice.

Turnips a close relative of cabbage, turnip leaves contain more calcium than any other vegetable. Turnip tops are an excellent source of this mineral that is especially needed by children for healthy bones and teeth, and by women to prevent osteoporosis (weak and brittle bones). Turnip leaves are an ideal, if surprising calcium-rich alternative to dairy produce and the raw leaves can be liquidised and blended with carrot juice for a highly nutritious drink, or steamed as a vegetable serving. Turnip tops are also an excellent source of beta carotene, vitamin C, B vitamins, magnesium, sulphur, iodine and iron. Be aware though, that 90 per cent of these nutrients are found in the turnip tops as opposed to its more common root.

The Nightshade Family

Tomatoes, aubergines, potatoes, and peppers are some of our most popular vegetables so it is perhaps surprising to learn that they are related to the deadly nightshade family. This is why these vegetables are avoided by macrobiotics who regard them all as mildly poisonous. It is also worth noting that those with arthritis and joint problems may find their condition improves if they stop eating vegetables from this family, especially tomatoes.

Although modern nutrition does not recognise the significance of the unique yin and yang values observed by macrobiotics, it does confirm that aubergines and potatoes contain high levels of alkaloids. These are alkaline substances mixed with nitrogen that are toxic at high doses. Even at low doses, alkaloids appear able to disrupt the metabolism in a similar way to caffeine. However, there is little scientific evidence that eating either tomatoes, aubergines, potatoes or peppers does the body much harm, so whether you choose to eat them or not is a personal decision.

Potatoes the main problem with potatoes occurs when the tubers are exposed to warm, light environments, such as under fluorescent supermarket lights. This encourages them to develop the most toxic form of alkaloids called solanine and chaconine. Fortunately, this process also produces chlorophyll which turns them green as a warning to us not to eat them. Solanine in particular causes headaches, nausea and stomach upsets and in high doses can result in brain disturbances. Solanine has also been inconclusively linked to spina bifida, where there is an incomplete closure of the spine in newborns. Incidents of potato blight in Ireland reduced crops to such an extent that green potatoes were eaten in larger quantities, while at the same time a rise in spina bifida babies was recorded. These powerful alkaloids are not destroyed by cooking so green potatoes should be avoided in the first place. Aubergines also contain *solanine* (their botanical name is *Solanum melongena*). In addition, potatoes tend to contain large amounts of contaminants and despite washing, peeling and boiling for 20 minutes, about 10 per cent of pesticide residue levels can still be detected in an average potato. This figure is even higher for potatoes baked in their skins, so it is well worth baking only organic varieties.

According to a 1988 report published in the *British Medical Journal*, there is also an association between all types of potato and sugar consumption and acute appendicitis, although the authors point out that this may be due to potatoes being eaten in place of other healthier green, leafy vegetables. Do remember, though, that potatoes have plenty of fibre (if eaten with their skins) and are a useful source of vitamin C. The best way to eat potatoes is either baked or boiled in their skins (a serving of chips has three times the calories and twelve times the fat of a baked potato). Raw potato juice is also said to be a useful internal cleanser and its soothing action is used by naturopaths to help stomach ulcers. It tastes disgusting but can be disguised by mixing it with carrot juice, or adding it to soups and sauces just before serving.

Tomatoes if you choose to eat potatoes and tomatoes it is especially important that both have been organically grown. The US National Research Council has found that the pesticides commonly found in tomatoes have the greatest potential for causing cancer. In addition, tomatoes are a relatively common culprit of food intolerance and can trigger skin rashes. Tomatoes contain substances called lectins which are also found in other foods such as wheat and beans, but which are usually destroyed by cooking. However, as most tomatoes are eaten raw they retain their high lectin content. While more research is needed, we do know that they can disrupt the function of the small intestine and may provoke psoriasis. Lectins also bind to connective tissue sheaths and muscle fibres and may be a factor in the disrupted and stiffened tissues that cause osteo- and rheumatoid arthritis. It may be a coincidence, but many arthritis sufferers specifically report that their symptoms subside when they stop eating tomatoes. But it is not all gloomy news for the tomato, as it is a very good source of beta carotene. However, most tomatoes are picked while still green and ripened by gassing with ethylene (a synthetic form of plant hormone) and gassed tomatoes have fewer nutrients than those that have been ripened naturally.

Peppers these were misnamed by Christopher Columbus in his search for peppercorns. They are also known by their botanical name *Capsicum* and are fruits from plants of the deadly nightshade family. Peppers are a good source of beta carotene, with red and yellow peppers containing more of this nutrient than the green. Peppers also have plenty of vitamin C (red and yellow peppers contain four times more vitamin C than oranges) and some potassium. If you choose to eat them, diced raw peppers are a colourful way of adding vitamins to a salad. Whole peppers are also delicious baked with a rice or lentil stuffing, although you lose most of the vitamin C by cooking them.

Luscious Lettuce And Other Green Leaves

Lettuce the Ancient Greeks loved lettuce and served it at the beginning and end of every meal. Salads made with lettuce leaves have been popular in Britain since the Middle Ages and in the 1700s French physicians said that salad should be eaten at the end of every meal 'to encourage sleep, free the stomach and temper the ardours of Venus'. Wild lettuce which has a milky white juice contains narcotic substances and has been used by herbalists for centuries as a sedative. This is probably why Peter Rabbit fell asleep in Mr McGregor's garden after feasting on his tender lettuces. Lettuce is reputedly good for the scalp. American herbalist Dr William Lee recommends a daily glass of lettuce and carrot juice to stimulate hair growth and prevent greying.

Lettuce is a reasonable source of some vitamins and minerals (see page 125) and again the darker the leaves, the more nutrients they contain. While iceberg is the most popular variety, it has the least to offer nutritionally. All lettuces should be washed thoroughly and, at the risk of sounding repetitive, be organically grown. According to the US National Research Council, lettuce is one of the main sources of unwanted nitrates in our diet. One study carried out by The Food Commission found that British lettuce contains, on average, 10 g of nitrates per kg of lettuce – two and a half times the legal limit allowed in Switzerland. One unfortunate specimen tested showed pesticide residues at *nineteen times* the Swiss Government's maximum levels. So much for salad being a healthy option.

Dandelion another even more nutritious salad leaf is the dandelion, honoured by early French herbalists who likened its powers to the tooth of a lion, hence its name, *dent de lion*. Dandelion leaves are rich in beta carotene, vitamin C, contain more iron than spinach and have useful amounts of calcium. Dandelion leaves also act as a mild laxative and tonic for the bladder, kidneys and liver. Young shoots can be added to salads and the older leaves are delicious steamed or lightly fried in a little olive oil. If growing dandelions, the plants can be covered with a plant pot or bucket to blanch the leaves and take away some of their bitterness. Dandelion roots can also be used to make a nutritious coffee substitute. The roots of two-year-old plants should be dug up in the autumn when they are well stocked with essential food reserves. Wipe the roots before baking them in a cool oven until dry. For the freshest 'coffee' taste, store the roots whole and grind into a powder just before using as you would instant coffee.

Spinach this is another leaf vegetable that can be served raw in salads. One of our most important B vitamins, folic acid, was first identified in spinach and is especially important during pregnancy as it guards against spina bifida and anencephaly, in which the brain fails to develop fully. Researchers at the University of Alabama's medical school have also established a link between folic acid and the prevention of cervical cancer. Although spinach is rich in iron (remember Popeye?) it also contains high levels of oxalic acid which make it difficult to absorb. This is because the oxalic acid combines with magnesium and calcium to carry it out of the body. However, spinach is an excellent source of the antioxidant beta carotene.

Watercress the Romans first used watercress leaves as a medicine, not a food, and one of its uses was as a hair tonic. Scientists have since learnt that watercress contains more sulphur than any other vegetable, apart from horseradish, and that sulphur-containing amino acids are important for healthy hair growth. Watercress also contains calcium, iron, B vitamins, vitamin C and iodine. Watercress leaves can be made into a juice and mixed with other vegetable juices to make a highly nutritious and tasty drink.

Green leaf lore

Nutrients per 4 oz (100 g)

Variety	Beta carotene iu	Vitamin C mg	Calcium mg	Iron mg
Iceberg	33	4	19	0.5
Butterhead	2600	24	68	1.4
Chicory	4000	24	100	0.9
Watercress	4700	43	120	0.2
Spinach	6700	28	100	2.7
Argula/ roquette	7400	91	68	1.4
Dandelion	14000	35	187	3.1

Source: University of California, Berkeley

Superb Salad Vegetables

Salads (in the widest sense) are the perfect way to add raw vegetables to your normal diet and just about any variety can be included. Try grating raw beetroot, Brussels sprouts, carrot and cabbage over a handful of mixed lettuce leaves, top with a few alfalfa sprouts, sunflower seeds and a herb dressing. More salad and dressing ideas can be found on pages 175–182, meanwhile, here are some of the best ingredients.

Avocado technically a fruit because it contains a seed, the avocado is native to Peru. It is a unique fruit because half its weight is made from natural oil. Fortunately, this oil is mono-unsaturated which means it is beneficial to the body and can even reduce cholesterol. Studies in California show that those who ate a low-fat diet with added avocados had lower cholesterol levels than those who ate a low-fat diet alone. After three weeks of an avocado-enriched diet testers had an average reduction in serum cholesterol of 8.2 per cent, whereas those who ate the low-fat diet alone dropped by just 4.9 per cent.

The oil in avocados is especially nourishing for the skin as it contains a high percentage of the skin's own internal moisturiser called linoleic acid. Avocados are also a useful source of potassium, vitamin B3 (niacin), vitamin E, beta carotene and iron. Avocados should be eaten when fully ripe and slightly soft to the touch (ripe avocados contain three times as much beta carotene as unripe fruits). To prevent half an avocado from discolouring, store it in the fridge with the stone intact and sprinkle a little lemon juice on the flesh.

Beetroot this vegetable developed from a sprawling plant that grew around the shores of the Caspian Sea. Originally only its leaves were eaten. The first recipes for the root date back to fifteenth century English cooking. According to the Doctrine of Signatures (the ancient herbal tome) which suggests that every plant reveals its original purpose by its shape or by colour (i.e. resembling the organ it can heal), beetroot was supposed to be good for the blood. It certainly contains some iron as well as calcium, potassium and magnesium. Beetroot is also a good source of beta carotene and vitamin C. The best way to cook beetroot is to bake it in its skin (see Baked Beetroot page 196). Raw beetroot is also good grated into salads or made into juice and mixed with carrot juice for a revitalising tonic.

Celeriac this bulbous white root vegetable is a hybrid of celery, hence its name. It is also known simply as celery root. Celeriac is a useful source of vitamin C and is delicious raw. Crisp, crunchy and stringless, celariac is a perfect ingredient for salads and home-made coleslaw.

Cucumber this vegetable belongs to the *Cucurbitaceae* family, along with pumpkins and marrows. The cucumber originated in India where it was heralded as a symbol of fertility. One Buddhist legend tells of an emperor's wife who had 60 000 offspring and the first was a cucumber which climbed to heaven on its own vine! Cucumber has a high water content and contains some vitamin C, potassium and other trace elements such as silicon and sulphur. It is a useful diuretic and helps flush water from the system and prevent water retention. As cucumbers are often waxed to preserve their shelf life they should be peeled before eating, unless organic varieties are available.

Fennel brought to Britain by the Romans, bunches of fennel were hung outside houses in medieval times to ward off witches. All parts of the plant can be eaten including the bulb, stalk and seeds and they have faintly aniseed flavours. Fennel is a natural digestive and the crushed seeds are used in gripe water to soothe infant colic. The natural oils in fennel are a good contrast to fatty foods such as pork and mackerel, and are said to soothe an irritated stomach. Fennel may be lightly steamed or eaten raw and is also reputed to have a mild diuretic action.

Mushrooms cultivated mushrooms contain traces of iron, B vitamins and potassium. Don't pick wild mushrooms unless you know *exactly* what to look for as many varieties are highly poisonous. All fungi, including wild mushrooms, should be avoided by those with *candidiasis* (thrush) as the spores can aggravate this fungal condition. Mushrooms should be wiped with a clean, damp cloth before eating and stored in a paper bag or open container in the fridge.

Radish rich in vitamin C, the radish was named from the Anglo-Saxon word *rude*, meaning red. However, it has been around for far longer and pictures of radishes are carved on the walls of the Egyptian temples at Karnack. There was even a solid gold statue of a radish in the temple at Delphi. Radishes are rich in the *amyclytic* enzyme which is useful in urinary tract disorders and is said to prevent gallstones. They are also strongly alkaline which is supposed to benefit the kidneys and bladder. If you cut a radish four or six times almost to the base and place in a bowl of ice-cold water it will open up like a flower. The Japanese white radish or *daikon* looks more like a large white carrot but has an interesting spicy flavour. It is especially good cut into strips for crudités, or grated into salads.

Remarkable Root Vegetables

Burdock this blackened root is one of our most powerful internal cleansers and is a rich source of skin-strengthening sulphur, iron and B vitamins. It is high in insulin which helps stabilise blood sugars and may be helpful for diabetics. It also contains several anti-fungal and anti-bacterial substances. Burdock was probably first used in tenth-century Japan as a convalescent food to speed recovery from illness. Herbalists have used burdock for centuries as an effective kidney and liver tonic as it stimulates the production of bile and helps the elimination processes. Burdock is specifically said to help the colon throw off excess sticky mucus and is a useful ingredient of a de-tox diet. Herbalists also use extract of burdock to cleanse a spotty or irritated skin from within, and it may also help eczema and dermatitis. An unusual root vegetable, fresh burdock roots can sometimes be found in some health food shops and from organic produce suppliers. Otherwise, it may be bought dried or in the form of liquid tinctures from shops that stock herbal remedies. Fresh burdock can be cooked or used raw in the same way as carrots or parsnips. It is especially good for stir-fried dishes.

Carrots the British we have a particular passion for carrots and Britain is the largest worldwide consumer per person of carrots. We each eat, on average, 9 kg (20 lb) of carrots every year. An important group of vitamins called the carotenoids were so called because they were first found in carrots. These include one of our most important nutrients, beta carotene. According to the American cancer specialist Dr Freudenheim, the risks of cancer are substantially reduced by eating even a modest amount of fruit and vegetables. He says, 'eating a carrot a day would raise beta carotene levels sufficiently to give considerable protection'. Carrots are also reputed to help us see in the dark and their beta carotene content is needed for healthy eyes as well as clear skin.

Carrots belong to the *Umbelliferae* family and this word comes from the latin for 'umbrella' because of the plant's parasol top of flowers. Their attractive foliage earned carrots the nickname 'Queen Anne's lace' and in the fourteenth century Dutch noblewomen wore the feathery leaves in their hair. There are over 3000 species in this family, including the herbs dill, coriander, cumin, caraway and parsley. As most of a carrot's nutrients lie just beneath the surface they should be scrubbed, not peeled. They are one of our most versatile vegetables and can be served raw in salads or chopped into sticks for crudités. Carrots are also easy to juice and their naturally high sugar content makes grated carrot a tasty addition to home-made bread, muffins and carrot cake. If used as a cooked vegetable, carrots should be lightly steamed and are especially good served with arame seaweed (see page 136), parsnips or broccoli.

Parsnip this close relative of the carrot used to be a staple of the British diet before being largely replaced by the potato in the nineteenth century. A useful source of vitamin C, parsnips have been used for centuries as a diuretic, anti-arthritic and de-tox agent. They contain a rare combination of sulphur and silicon which is especially useful for strengthening weak nails and brittle hair. Parsnips have a sweet, nutty flavour and are delicious baked in their skins or puréed with a little mashed carrot.

Salsify an unusual carrot-shaped, root vegetable that can have a black or white skin depending on the variety. Both types contain vitamin C, calcium and iron. Salsify should be steamed whole before peeling and slicing, and it tastes like asparagus.

Perfect Pods

There are several thousand varieties of beans and peas which all belong to the *legume* family. Legumes are unusual vegetables as they contain 17–25 per cent protein, roughly double that of wholegrains. They also have useful amounts of iron, potassium, calcium, beta carotene, vitamin C and vitamin B3 (niacin). Dried beans and peas are known as pulses and these are a staple part of many diets worldwide (see pages 72–4).

Peas are the oldest legume and are thought to have been grown in the Garden of Eden, between the Euphrates and the Tigris river. Remains of peas have also been found in the ruins of Troy and the pre-dynastic Egyptian tombs. In Europe, peas found at a Swiss neolithic lake village have been carbon dated as far back as 4500 BC. Although beans can be traced back almost as far, they have a checkered history. Broad beans were thought to be 'unclean' by Egyptian priests and the Romans only used them as counters in elections. In Italy broad beans were only ever eaten after a funeral, hence the expression 'bean feast'.

Broad beans have a good supply of calcium and iron and fresh bean juice has been used to treat fatigue. Runner beans are also particularly high in calcium and are a rare source of a B vitamin called inositol which plays a part in regulating cholesterol. Fresh, dried or tinned, legumes are also an excellent source of fibre. Frozen peas are also one of the few vegetables that can taste better when frozen as they are frozen within hours of picking. Frozen peas and beans are useful for throwing into instant stir-frys or for adding colour and flavour to a risotto and other vegetable dishes. Petits pois are not a special variety, but are peas that have been picked very young and have a lower natural sugar content. They have a French name because they were first eaten by the court of king Louis XIV. The fresh or frozen flat pea pods called mange tout (also developed in France) are another tasty source of vitamins and fibre. Try them lightly steamed and added to salads or stir-fried.

Know Your Onions

Spring onions, chives, leeks and garlic belong to the same family and all are reputed to cleanse the system with their unique anti-bacterial properties. Highly versatile cooking ingredients, they can be added to almost every savoury dish for an extra flavour.

Onions onions contain the naturally antiseptic oils allyl disulphate and cycloallin, and researchers at the Royal Victoria Infirmary in Newcastle have found that cycloallin helps the walls of blood vessels (especially veins) dissolve clots which form inside them. This useful substance even seems to resist high temperatures, including frying. Onions also have beta carotene, potassium and the sulphur-containing amino acid cysteine. Unfortunately, most conventional crops of onions are also sprayed with chemical anti-sprouting agents.

Onions, spring onions and shallots are essential ingredients in many savoury recipes. They can be peeled under water to avoid tears, or peeled before chopping off the root end, as it is the root that releases the irritating fumes. The most powerful member of this family of plant healers is undoubtedly garlic, which is examined more closely in chapter six (pages 156–7).

Leeks these relatives of the onion are especially rich in potassium and can help eliminate uric acid from the system. This means that they are good foods for those suffering from gout and arthritis. The name leek is derived from *loch*, a word the Romans used to describe a cure for a sore throat. The Roman emperor Nero is reputed to have eaten a bowl of leek soup a day to improve his speaking voice. The Romans brought leeks to Britain where they have been popular for two thousand years. When the Welsh went into battle against the Saxons in AD 640, King Cadwallader's soldiers wore a leek to distinguish themselves from the English who had dressed in the same uniforms. Wales won the battle and the leek was adopted as a national emblem and is still worn on St David's day. Leeks contain fewer pungent oils than onions so are easier to slice without tears. They are best lightly steamed or stir-fried.

The Super Shoots

Artichoke the globe artichoke is a member of the daisy family and its edible heart contains protein, calcium, iron and potassium. Artichokes also contain the substance insulin that helps regulate sugars and carbohydrates. They were a particular favourite with King Henry VIII, who declared them to be an aphrodisiac. Artichokes are traditionally served as appetisers and have been found to contain a substance called cynarine which stimulates the flow of bile in the liver. This substance can also spark liver cell regeneration and is used to treat liver problems, including jaundice. Few appetisers are more nutritious or easier to prepare than lightly steamed artichokes served with a drizzle of walnut oil and a squeeze of lemon juice. For the best results, cook them in a covered pan with an inch of water so that the stem is softened by the boiling water while the leaves are lightly steamed.

Asparagus the reason why asparagus is so expensive is that it takes several years before a plant can be harvested. Asparagus is a member of the lily family and is unusual because it has both male and female plants. Despite being a slow starter, once established, asparagus spears can grow rapidly. Individual spears have been known to grow as much as 25 cm (10 inch) a day!

In addition to its delicious taste that has driven gourmets wild the world over, asparagus is an excellent source of beta carotene, vitamin C and contains some vitamin E and iron. It also contains the bioflavanoid rutin that helps strengthen the tiny capillaries in the skin. Raw asparagus contains an alkaloid called aspargine which stimulates the kidneys and is a powerful diuretic. Asparagus should be lightly cooked by steaming, or in the microwave oven for just a couple of minutes, and eaten while still slightly crisp. Its cooking water can also be saved and drunk as a diuretic, but as asparagus is high in purines it should be avoided altogether by those suffering from gout. Cooked, cooled asparagus is also an unusual addition to salads or cold dishes, and the tips make an attractive garnish for pasta or rice recipes.

Celery this shoot vegetable has a high water content and contains some vitamin C and a few other trace minerals. It is closely related to parsley and both are used by herbalists as a diuretic and natural laxative. Celery also contains plant hormones and essential oils which give it its distinctive smell. Celery juice is used by herbalists to balance the nervous system and is even reputed to restore a flagging sex drive. Fresh celery is full of fibre and gives extra 'crunch' to salads and coleslaw.

Terrific Tubers And Squash

Courgettes and marrow both these vegetables contain beta carotene, vitamin C, vitamin B (niacin) and potassium. They should be stored in the fridge and used within a week. Courgettes should be crisp and tender and can be eaten raw. Try cutting them into strips for crudités or grating them into salads. Marrows are larger and are much tougher and need to be steamed or baked before eating. Marrows are especially good served with a lentil or wholegrain stuffing.

Jerusalem artichokes these knobbly tubers are ideal alternatives to potatoes as they contain a high percentage of starch. Jerusalem artichokes are one of the tastiest tubers and come from a plant related to the sunflower that was first cultivated by the North American Indians. Women from the Iroquois tribe were so fond of these tasty tubers that they were nicknamed 'the artichoke eaters'. Artichokes were later exported to Europe and first reached the shores of Italy where they were called *girasole* (meaning sunflower), later misinterpreted by the British as 'Jerusalem' artichokes.

Spaghetti squash this yellow vegetable is shaped like a rugby ball and belongs to the same family as marrow, pumpkin and other squashes. It gets its name from its stringy fibrous inside that can be served instead of spaghetti. It is especially good for those who like their pasta sauce but want to avoid wheat. To cook it cut it in half and boil in a large pan of water for 20–30 minutes. You then use a fork to scrape out the fibrous strands before serving. Spaghetti squash is a good source of beta carotene, B vitamins and potassium.

Sweet potatoes these starchy tubers are not related to potatoes although they can be used in the same way. Sweet potatoes are the tuberous root of a vine related to morning glory and are native to Peru. Sweet potatoes are also incorrectly known as yams, which belong to the tropical *Discorea* family. They do look very similar and the confusion arose when African slaves used their own word *nyam* for the sweet potato when taken to America. Sweet potatoes are a useful source of beta carotene and contain some calcium and iron. They are also an excellent source of vitamin C and should be cooked with their skins intact to preserve their nutrients. Baked sweet potatoes need about twice the cooking time of ordinary potatoes. It is best to put them in a covered casserole dish as the natural sugars can cause the tubers to burst open. Their natural sweetness makes them especially popular with babies and children.

Vegetables From The Sea

Seaweeds are some of the oldest vegetables known to mankind and they were used extensively by the Ancient Greeks, Chinese and Roman dynasties. There are over 1700 species of seaweed, including kelp which is commonly taken as a nutritious food supplement. Seaweeds are rich in thirteen vitamins (notably vitamins C, D, beta carotene and several B vitamins) and contain twenty amino acids. Seaweed is also a good source of vitamin B12, which is important for non-meat eaters as there are few non-animal sources of this vitamin. Their high vitamin and mineral content also make seaweeds valuable organic fertilisers that dramatically enrich the soil.

Seaweeds contain large amounts of iodine, needed for the thyroid gland to regulate the metabolism and help weight control. Even a small shortage of iodine can induce nervous tension and insomnia, and the chlorine used to disinfect our water supply removes iodine from tap water. Iodine also has the unusual ability of protecting the body to some extent against radioactivity, including nuclear fallout. Seaweeds also contain alginic acid which binds with heavy metals such as lead within the body and removes them from the system.

These nutritional giants are the largest plants in the world, larger even than the Californian Redwood trees. Pacific kelps measure over 152 metres (500 feet) long and grow at the staggering rate of 30 cm (1 foot) per day.

The only nationality to use seaweeds extensively as foods today are the Japanese, who use them in soups, sauces and wrapped round rice rolls or raw fish to make sushi. American Health Foundation research suggests that the low rates of cancer amongst the Japanese (notably breast cancer) may have something to do with their high intake of seaweed. The Samurai warriors of Japan also used seaweed as bandages and today seaweed extracts are used in many modern dressings as they help blood to clot. Although we may not realise it, the British also consume a great deal of seaweed extracts which are added in the form of thickeners to ice-creams, beers, toothpaste, jellies, pies and puddings.

Many forms of dried seaweed can be found in health food shops and they are very economical to use. Instructions on the packet explain how to prepare and cook the various seaweeds. A small packet goes a long way and will last for many years if kept cool and dry. Unfortunately, sea vegetables are as susceptible to pollution as those grown on land, so note their country of origin. The least polluted waters for harvesting seaweeds are around the tip of Brittany, in Alaska and Japan. Seaweeds from the polluted waters of the North Sea, most of the English Channel, the Mediterranean and the Baltic should be avoided. Many of the more interesting and unusual varieties, such as *arame* and *hiziki*, are imported directly from Japan and can be found in speciality food shops.

Agar agar sold in the form of flakes or threads made by freeze-drying red Japanese seaweed called *tengusa*. Agar-agar contains alginates which are powerful gelling agents that gel at 50°C so dishes stay set even in very hot weather. It is a good non-animal alternative to gelatine which often contains additives.

Arame with a mild flavour, these thin strips can be soaked and added to noodles or mixed with other vegetables. Arame is especially good cooked and served with diced carrots.

Dulse a traditional Irish sea vegetable, this purple-coloured seaweed is rich in iron and has a slightly spicy flavour. It is easy to prepare and requires brief soaking before being added to soups, salads and vegetable dishes.

Hiziki these glistening black strips of seaweed are rich in many minerals and have a strong flavour. Known in Japan as 'bearer of wealth and beauty', hiziki is an acquired taste. Try serving it with stir-fried tofu and roasted sesame seeds or cook the strips in boiling water and use instead of spaghetti. Hiziki is especially rich in calcium and iron.

Kombu also known as kelp, this thick brown plant is a very valu-able cooking ingredient. Kelp contains glutamic acid, a part of monosodium glutamate (MSG), and gives a delicious flavour to soups, stocks and sauces. Slices of kombu cooked with beans and pulses also help to tenderise them by softening their fibres. This reduces their cooking time, makes them more digestible and reduces flatulence or wind. Powdered kelp is also available as a flavoursome thickener for soups and sauces.

Nori one of the tastiest of all sea vegetables, nori is sold in thin square sheets for wrapping around rice balls (or simply eating on its own as a highly nutritious snack). Cook sweet brown rice and serve it wrapped in the nori. You can tuck a spoonful of Japanese pickle or a cube of marinated tofu in the middle of the rice for a healthy fast food snack. Shredded nori is also available for sprink-ling on soups and salads. Nori is extremely high in iron and beta carotene – no kitchen should be without it!

Wakame this is another great flavour-enhancer and tenderiser as it also contains glutamic acid. A close relative of kelp, both are rich in iodine although wakame has a milder flavour. Wakame should be pre-soaked before adding to broths such as the traditional Japanese miso soup.

POWERFUL PLANT OILS

Eat yourself beautiful with one tablespoonful each day. The powers of natural plant oils are legendary. Olive oil was one of the first oils known to man and was used as a medicine, food, beauty treatment, fuel for lamps and even as a form of currency. It was so precious that Homer described it as 'liquid gold' and it has long been a symbol of strength, peace and fertility. Huge copper casks of olive oil were found buried beside the pharoahs in their pyramid tombs and it was highly prized for Egyptian sacrificial ceremonies. Galen, one of the first physicians, used olive oil to soothe sunburned skin and Hippocrates recommended it for stomach ulcers. Hippocrates used many plant oils in his treatments, including linseed oil which he prescribed for stomach and skin disorders. Sesame oil also has an illustrious history and can be traced back to Roman times. This versatile cooking oil was commonly used in Roman cooking and was first brought to Britain in AD 43. Other parts of the world used different oils according to their local crops. In South America the Aztecs pulverised sunflower seeds to extract a golden oil, while Mediterranean countries chose nut oils pressed from almonds, hazelnuts and

139

walnuts. Plant oils have a long and important history in preserving our health and it is a mistake to neglect their benefits today.

The Importance Of Plant Oils

Oils are generally extracted from nuts, seeds and wholegrains. These kernels contain the concentrated goodness needed for a plant to germinate and grow. They are the lifeforce of the plant and have unique health and beauty benefits. Plant oils are an amazingly rich source of some vitamins, minerals and nutrients called essential fatty acids (EFAs). These substances are required by every living cell in the body to function. EFAs make up the lipids, or fats, that surround all cells. Without an adequate supply of EFAs our cells become weak and vulnerable to attack by free radicals. EFAs are also especially important to strengthen the outer membrane surrounding skin cells. This protective shield helps skin cells to resist premature ageing and keeps the skin supple and strong. There is no doubt that strengthening our skin from within is one of the most fundamental aspects of a clear, glowing complexion.

Can Perfect Skin Be Created?

Yes! The most effective way to encourage a better looking complexion is not with an expensive skin-care regime but with the simple nutrients the skin demands in order to work properly. We make our own skin – it does not come out of a jar. The fundamental principle is to provide the skin with the basic ingredients it needs from within. These ingredients include EFAs, vitamin E and lecithin. We need small amounts of these substances so our skin can glow with good health. If our food lacks these nutrients our skin is often the first to suffer. One sign that we are low in essential fatty acids is dry, chapped or irritated skin. This occurs when cell membranes are weakened and the skin is unable to preserve its lipid barrier that prevents internal moisture from escaping. Fortunately, there is an easy answer as unrefined plant oils, such as olive oil or sunflower oil are especially rich in EFAs, vitamin E and lecithin. A tablespoonful taken every day is the best possible form of internal moisturiser and a powerful weapon to fight the signs of skin ageing and wrinkles.

Linoleic acid one of the main components of strong, healthy skin is linoleic acid, an EFA that is part of the skin cell membrane. This substance also forms the protective lipid barrier that locks moisture into the skin. Linoleic acid is also the parent of another EFA called gamma linolenic acid (GLA). This is used for many metabolic processes and is especially useful for skin disorders such as eczema.

Vitamin E an essential nutrient for healthy skin (see page 21 for the richest sources). A powerful antioxidant, vitamin E neutralises the damage caused by free radicals within the skin. This is especially important when it comes to preventing the signs of premature ageing, such as fine lines and wrinkles. Vitamin E also strengthens the tiny capillary walls and encourages the larger blood vessels to dilate or widen. This reduces blood pressure and allows an increased flow of blood to deliver essential oxygen supplies to the skin cells.

Lecithin this strengthens cell membranes. Lecithin is one of the many substances that make up the cocktail of compounds called Natural Moisturising Factors (NMFs) found in the skin. NMFs are powerful internal moisturisers and work by absorbing moisture from the atmosphere and holding on to it within the skin. Lecithin also functions as a kind of edible detergent that breaks up large fat deposits, such as cholesterol, so they can be more easily removed from the body. For this reason, lecithin may be one of the many dietary keys to solving the problem of heart disease.

Skin Strengtheners

Plant oils are the richest source of these skin strengthening nutrients and a small amount should be added to our diet every day. Just one tablespoonful of unrefined cooking oil is enough to nourish and fortify our skin cells from within. It is important that they are high quality, cold-pressed or unrefined oils as these still retain their nutrients. Refined cooking oils have had their natural nutrients stripped away and may also contain traces of the chemical hexane used in the extraction process. Plant oils are either monounsaturated (e.g. olive and sesame oil) or polyunsaturated (e.g. sunflower and safflower oil) and nutritionists say that they should form one per cent of our diet. A tiny amount, but enough to supply our cells with the vital oils they need to flourish. However, there is one snag: despite our high-fat diet, most of us eat the *wrong type* of fats, so probably don't even get the tiny amount of vital oils we need.

The Fat Factor

Despite their bad press, not all oils and fats are harmful. The good guys are the natural plant oils, such as olive oil, that contain the nutrients the body must have in order to thrive. These are easy to recognise as they are always liquid at room temperature. The bad guys are the saturated fats that clog our arteries, encourage weight gain and are a factor in causing cancer. Saturated fats are almost always animal in origin and tend to be solid when at room temperature.

As mentioned briefly in chapter one, the other fats that should be avoided are the hydrogenated fats. Hydrogenation is the process that hardens a liquid vegetable oil into a solid fat so that is can be used in processed foods. The technique is widely used to convert sunflower oil and other oils into low-fat spreads. However, when an oil is hydrogenated or hardened it loses its healthy properties and behaves like a saturated fat in the body. This means that any product containing hydrogenated vegetable oil may not be as healthy as it appears. The intensive heating required for the hydrogenation process has another side-effect too. It converts the structure of linoleic acid and other healthy 'cis-fatty acids' into more dangerous 'trans-fatty acids'. These interfere with cellular activity and block the health-giving benefits of other essential fatty acids. It is worth looking for un-hydrogenated low-fat spreads available from health food shops or choosing soft spreads that have fewer trans-fatty acids than hardened margarines.

For many years we have been told the virtues of a low-fat diet and, to a great extent, this message is very sound. However, in cutting out the harmful saturated fats we must not ignore the beneficial oils that the body needs. The nutrients in oils are called essential fatty acids for a very good reason: they are essential for life. The body cannot make its own supplies but must obtain them only through food. Not only do the EFAs surround the membrane of every cell in the body, but they also make up the fat that surrounds our internal organs. This layer of cushioning acts as important shock-absorption and protective insulation. Many EFAs have roles in areas of active tissue functioning, for example, in the brain and sense organs. One tablespoonful of unrefined plant oil used in cooking every day is the perfect way to make sure your body benefits.

Evening Primrose Oil

Oils such as evening primrose oil and fish oils have been used successfully to treat diseases as diverse as heart disease, multiple sclerosis, eczema and psoriasis. The EFAs found in these oils make a number of biological regulators called prostaglandins. These control communications between cells and although scientists have yet to pinpoint exactly how prostaglandins work, we do know that they have a role in just about everything and anything that goes on inside us. Prostaglandins are made on the spot depending on where they are needed and live for only a fraction of a second. This is why it is so important to keep up a daily intake of EFAs to provide a steady supply of the raw material needed to create them.

The EFA called linoleic acid is found in plant oils as well as being present to a lesser extent in fruits, wholegrains and vegetables. Once inside the body, some linoleic acid is converted into GLA. GLA is a rare substance and is only available from a few other natural sources, principally breast milk, borage oil and evening primrose oil. GLA is needed for its specific anti-inflammatory action and it is converted into the prostaglandin known as PGE1. This substance controls inflammation and activates the T-lymphocytes that are part of our immune system. It also helps to prevent the abnormal cell turnover that causes many severe skin conditions and is the reason why GLA is so important for anyone suffering from eczema, psoriasis or dermatitis.

In theory, the body should make enough of its own GLA from linoleic acid in the diet, but many factors interfere with the conversion process. These include saturated fats in the diet, smoking and other forms of pollution, stress and some medications. Those who feel their skin is suffering should limit these factors, add more plant oils to their food and take a daily supplement of borage or evening primrose oil both rich in GLA. Medically proven, evening primrose oil is even available now on prescription for the treatment of eczema and breast pain, and many women with pre-menstrual syndrome also find it helpful.

Fish Oils For Brain And Bones

In addition to the EFAs found in plant oils there is another group of essential fatty acids found only in fish. These are made from the parent fatty acid called alpha linolenic acid, which remains liquid even at very cold temperatures and is found in large quantities in deep sea fish. These 'oily' fish include mackerel, herring and the livers of cod, hence cod liver oil. Alpha linolenic acid is converted by the body into two important EFAs known as EPA and DHA. These regulate blood fats throughout the body and are able to reduce cholesterol and keep the arteries clear. Fish oils are now available on prescription to treat heart disease and eating oily fish is recommended by nutritionists. EPA and DHA are also a vital part of brain functioning and are used by the foetus to develop healthy brain tissues, so oily fish or fish oil supplements may be a useful addition to a pregnant woman's diet. A study reported in *The Lancet* in April 1992 revealed that women who took a daily dose of fish oils gave birth to stronger, healthier babies. Scientists are also currently considering adding EPA and DHA to the feeds of premature babies who may not have received sufficient supplies before birth. Either way, modern research has managed to prove yet another old wives' tale that fish is indeed good for the brain.

In addition to helping combat heart disease and helping with brain development, fish oils have other specific benefits for the skin. The prostaglandins that are made from alpha linolenic acid help reduce the levels of inflammatory chemicals called leukotrienes. These are found in abnormally high levels in those with eczema and psoriasis and several clinical trials indicate that fish oil supplements may be helpful. Because they can help control inflammation, fish oils are also useful in many cases of rheumatoid arthritis. Cod liver oil has a medical licence to treat stiff joints and many elderly people swear by its powers to prevent pain and swelling. The EFAs converted from alpha linolenic acid may also be helpful in other cases of pain such as migraine and menstrual cramps that are caused by a build-up of inflammatory agents. Vegetarians or vegans who do not eat fish may risk a deficiency of these important nutrients. They can consider taking a linseed oil supplement which contains a version of alpha linolenic acid that acts in a slightly less effective, but similar, way within the body.

Cooking With Oils

Unrefined cooking oils are versatile cooking ingredients. Although more expensive than refined oils, they contain many more nutrients and are well worth the extra expense. Although most oils look the same on the shelves, many have very different characteristics. Olive oil, sesame seed oil, almond and hazelnut oil are all monounsaturated oils. Their chemical structure makes them the most stable at high temperatures and so these oils are by far the best to use for any recipe that needs heating. Personally, I only use olive oil for frying or any recipe that needs heating. Although the long-term hazards of heated polyunsaturated oils are unclear, it seems sensible to choose a cooking oil that withstands high temperatures. Once *any* oil has been heated to a high temperature, though, it should always be thrown away. Never re-use any oil that has been used for frying as its chemical structure breaks down with each heating to produce peroxides which form free radicals in the body. Any cooking oil that starts to smoke should also be discarded as this is a sign that its chemical structure has started to break down.

Polyunsaturated oils, such as sunflower, safflower or corn oil, should not be used at all for frying. This is because their chemical structure is easily broken down to produce toxic by-products that lead to the formation of free radicals. However, polyunsaturated oils do contain important EFAs and should be used in recipes which only need gentle heating or used cold in salad dressings. Never buy a blended oil unless you know exactly what is inside the bottle. Many are made with cheaply refined oils and can be of very low quality. Always read the label and make sure that the oil you are buying is unrefined. Olive oil usually has the words 'cold-pressed' written on the label if it is unrefined and is available from most supermarkets. Otherwise, most other oils are available in unrefined versions from health food shops.

COOKING OILS

Name	Culinary uses	Saturates %	Oleic %*	Linoleic %**
Corn	baking, dressings	12	25	57
Hazelnut	dressings, flavouring, frying	8	77	10
Olive	all, including deep-frying	14	70	10
Safflower	sauces, dressings	10	12	73
Sesame	sauces, dressings, flavouring	15	40	40
Sunflower	sauces, dressings	15	30	50
Walnut	dressings, flavouring	10	15	55

*Monounsaturated
**Polyunsaturated

The oils recommended in this chart are all available in unrefined form

THE VITAL COOKING OILS

Corn oil also known as maize oil, is extracted from sweetcorn kernels and is one of the cheapest oils available. High in polyunsaturates, it is possible to find unrefined corn oil in health food shops and this contains useful levels of vitamin E. Being polyunsaturated, corn oil deteriorates at high temperatures so it is best kept for using cold in dressings or gently warmed. Corn oil is a good base for an inexpensive salad dressing that can be mixed with a small amount of a more expensive oil, such as walnut or hazelnut for flavouring.

Grapeseed oil this is extracted from grape pips and so, not surprisingly, the highest producers are around the wine regions of France, Australia and California. Grapeseed oil has one of the highest contents of polyunsaturated fatty acids, second only to safflower, but is not generally available in an unrefined version. My bottle of grapeseed oil sits in the bathroom, not the kitchen, as it is a great base for massage oils. In fact, most aroma-therapists use grapeseed oil as their carrier oil for their fragrant essential oils as it is light, easily absorbed by the skin and does not leave a sticky trace on clothing.

Groundnut oil also known as peanut oil as it is extracted from peanut kernels. Technically, peanuts are not nuts at all but are seed pods from the *legume* family. In their raw state, peanuts are highly nutritious and contain about 45 per cent pure oil, 30 per cent protein and useful amounts of iron, vitamin E and B vitamins. However, refining the oil takes away these valuable nutrients and it can be hard to find peanut oil in an unrefined form. Similarly, dry roasted peanuts and other processed nut snacks may well contain rancid oils that are best avoided. If you want to add peanut oil to your diet, the best way is with a handful of freshly shelled peanuts.

Hazelnut oil high in monounsaturates, this comes from the Mediterranean where its production is very much a cottage industry. It is relatively easy to find unrefined versions. Most hazelnut oil is still extracted by hand processes that involve pressing the nuts between huge stone slabs and filtering the oil through muslin cloths. It is a labour-intensive business which accounts for its high price, matched only by walnut oil which is produced in a similar way. Hazelnut oil is highly versatile, being both safe to heat and a tasty addition to salad dressings. Its light texture and nutty flavour are also useful for baking and many a cake or biscuit mixture has been improved with a spoonful of this delicious oil. Hazelnut oil has the lowest saturated fat content of any cooking oil.

Olive oil there is no doubt that olive oil is a culinary superstar and that no kitchen should be without it. Mankind has cooked with olive oil for thousands of years and modern science has finally proved that the instincts of early civilisations were right to do so. One factor in the low rates of cancer and heart disease in Mediterranean countries is thought to be due to their passion for olive oil. A monounsaturated oil, olive oil is highly stable at high temperatures and one of the very best for cooking. It is easily available cold-pressed, which generally means that it is also unrefined. If in doubt, look at the colour of the oil. The darker the oil, the more natural nutrients have been left behind (the same is true of any cooking oil – always go for darker colours, except when the oil has been artificially 'toasted').

The label on an olive oil bottle reveals more about its contents than any other type of oil. Extra virgin olive oil comes from the first pressing of the olives and has the darkest, greenest colour. Extra virgin olive oil is also the most highly flavoured and has a pungent aroma that you either love or loathe. Most gourmets have a healthy addiction to it, which explains why extra virgin olive oil can cost as much as Champagne. The second pressing of the olives gives us virgin olive oil, which is also of extremely high quality and has an aromatic flavour. Virgin olive oil is the slightly cheaper of the two and, in my opinion, just as good. Beware of any olive oil that is simply labelled 'pure olive oil' as this means that it has been refined. It is paler in colour and does not have the same vitamin E and lecithin content as the others.

Olive oil is one of the few cooking oils that stores well and one of the most economical ways to buy it is in a large metal drum. It can be decanted into smaller glass bottles and stored tightly sealed in a cool, dark place. Those who are extremely health conscious can even store their olive oil in the fridge as the cold temperature causes the small saturated part of the oil to solidify and sink to the bottom of the bottle. When the oil has been finished the last inch or so of saturated fat crystals can be discarded.

Rapeseed oil this crop is a newcomer to the British landscape and its vivid yellow flowers are welcomed by some for their cheerfulness and cursed by others for their pollen that can bring on hay fever and asthma attacks. The rape plant is a brassica and its high-protein seed yields the vegetable oil, which is also known as canola oil by the Canadians. Rapeseed oil is cheap, high in both polyunsaturates and monounsaturates and has a light, versatile texture. However, it produces more toxic by-products than most when heated and so should not be used for frying. Unfortunately I have yet to find an unrefined version of rapeseed oil.

149

Safflower oil the safflower is related to the thistle and is now cultivated around the world for its useful oil. The oil is extracted from safflower seeds and is an excellent source of poly-unsaturated fatty acids. Although it should not be heated to high temperatures, it is excellent used cold in dressings and sauces. Safflower oil has a light, slightly nutty taste and is available in an unrefined form.

Sesame oil popular since Roman times, this oil is extracted from the seeds of the tall sesame plant. Sesame oil is monounsaturated and so may be safely heated. It is also available in an unrefined form from health food shops. Some varieties of sesame seed oil are also heated and sold as toasted sesame oil. This thick, black version is an essential ingredient in some Chinese cookery but as it contains a high level of damaging peroxides (which cause free radicals to form) it is not recommended for regular use.

Soybean oil this comes from the soya bean which is a member of the *legume* family. The soya bean is a remarkable plant that can be traced back over 5000 years to early cultivation in China. Although the soya bean itself is highly nutritious and rich in pro-tein, it contains less than 20 per cent plant oil. This makes extrac-tion difficult and means that manufacturers have to use a solvent extraction process involving the petrochemical hexane. When using unrefined soybean oil not only are you avoiding the hexane, but it is also providing you with a good source of vitamin E and it contains more lecithin than any other vegetable oil. As with other oils high in polyunsaturates it should not be heated to high tem-peratures.

Sunflower oil this popular cooking oil originated in Mexico and Peru where crops of sunflowers have been cultivated for thousands of years. Sunflower oil is extracted from the mass of seeds that make up the centre of the sunflower's head and they contain about 40 per cent pure oil. Sunflower oil is rich in polyun-saturates, has a mild, sweet flavour and is excellent for using cold or warm in many recipes. Unrefined sunflower oil is available from most health food shops and may be blended with one of the more expensive nut oils for a lighter texture and richer flavour.

Walnut oil a favourite with French chefs for centuries who even use walnut oil to fry eggs, a few drops can transform an ordinary salad dressing into something special. Walnut oil is increasingly available from supermarkets where it is sold in small fancy bottles with equally fancy price tags. For the best value, buy it direct from the mill if you go to France. Walnut oil is high in polyunsaturated fatty acids and is sometimes sold under its French name of *huile de noix,* or *huile de noix extra* which is the first pressing and has a stronger flavour.

STORING OILS

One problem with cooking oils is that they are highly susceptible to damage from heat, light and air. As soon as you take the top off and expose them to the atmosphere they start to deteriorate. Polyunsaturated oils are the most at risk of rancidity and should be stored in the fridge after opening. Monounsaturated oils such as olive oil can be stored in a cupboard, but all oils should be kept tightly sealed and out of the light. If possible, buy oils in metal containers or amber glass bottles which protect the oils during storage. Ideally, only buy oils in small quantities. It is far better to shop more often for oils than to have to use up a huge bottle of rancid oil that contains free radicals. However, unrefined oils do last longer than refined oils as they have not been stripped of their vitamin E which acts as an antioxidant and protects the oil from rancidity, but even so it is best to use them within weeks.

HEALING HERBS

Eat yourself beautiful with two varieties each day. Herbs are nature's own cure-alls and the art of herbalism was mankind's first form of medicine. Neanderthal man used medicinal herbs as far back as 60 000 years ago and traces of many species have been found in their burial sites. Some say that herbalism is still the most effective form of medicine and there are many practising herbalists in Britain today.

Certainly many modern medicines have herbal origins and scientists are only just beginning to understand some of their more unusual properties. For example, the foxglove gives us digitalis, a powerful medicine used in heart disease to stimulate the vagus nerve that keeps the heart beating; liquorice root has been used as an expectorant since Roman times and is still a common ingredient in cough medicines; morphine and codeine come from the opium poppy; aspirin comes from the white willow and slippery elm is one of the most effective treatments for stomach ulcers. In Tudor times, King Henry VIII issued a law to protect herbal medicine which was later reaffirmed in the 1968 British Medical Act. Herbs are popular worldwide and in the Far

East you are still more likely to be treated with these natural compounds than synthetic drugs. So great are the powers of these aromatic plants that entire encyclopaedias have been written about their properties and it takes many years to understand all their uses.

Basically, all herbs and spices owe their richly aromatic smells to a high concentration of essential oils used by the plant to store surplus energy. These oils have many unusual properties and all are highly anti-bacterial. These fragrant oils are also antioxidants and as such can neutralise the damage caused by destructive free radicals. Some herbs have additional benefits and may also be anti-fungal, anti-microbial and naturally antibiotic. Herbs are also a rich source of vitamins, minerals and trace elements. Parsley, for example, is one of our richest sources of vitamin C, and although we tend to eat herbs in tiny quantities, even small amounts will add up to better health.

Anti-Ageing Herbs

Many of the concentrated oils found in herbs have been recognised as powerful antioxidants for many years, but scientists have only recently proved their power to actually turn back the clock. Studies by the Scottish Agricultural College in association with researchers in Hungary have managed to pinpoint their dramatic effect on ageing. One of the first signs of the body ageing is deterioration of the membranes surrounding our cells. This makes it harder for cells to function effectively and occurs when the EFAs within the cell membrane are reduced. In skin cells, for example, this causes skin sagging and leads to deep facial lines and wrinkles. The process of cellular ageing occurs throughout the body and is the cause of many diseases associated with ageing, such as senile dementia and acute memory loss. Herbs, however, may have the ability to reduce this: in trials where mice were fed the volatile oils from several herbs there was a significant rejuvenation of their cells. In particular, levels of the EFAs

DHA and linolenic acid greatly increased. In some cases, more of these EFAs were found in the older mice than in mice far younger. The significance of this is that the cells in the older mice were able to continue functioning well into old age and the animals enjoyed a greatly improved quality of life.

While the results have yet to be replicated in humans, team leader Dr Stanley Deans suggests sprinkling a few herbs on food at every opportunity. One of the most powerful herbs tested was common thyme, but Dr Deans points out that as most culinary herbs contain these fragrant oils, they all have a similar effect. It doesn't seem to matter whether the herbs are fresh, dried or frozen, as the oils withstand most processing. However, as a general rule, the fresher and tastier the herb, the more active ingredients it contains.

Cooking With Herbs

Herbs had a practical role in history as natural food preservatives as well as flavourings. They were highly prized and many of the early sea voyages to discover the New World were made in an attempt to break the monopolies of the spice trade. Christopher Columbus was spurred on in his search for herbs and spices, and brought back cinnamon, cloves and nutmeg from the West Indies to break the cartels of the powerful Venetian and Arabian traders. Herbs have been used in British cooking for centuries and recipes from the court of Richard II in 1390 reveal the extensive use of parsley, ginger, mint, garlic, sage, cinnamon, thyme and pepper. One popular recipe was for herb fritters dipped in honey and salads often included a variety of fresh herb leaves.

Basil a sacred herb in India that is used to cleanse and purify. Reputedly good for headaches, a pot of this fragrant herb in the kitchen will deter flies. Fresh and dried basil is high in beta carotene, calcium and iron. Basil is used extensively in Italian cooking as it complements tomatoes, pasta and rich cheeses.

Bay these leaves come from an evergreen tree and have been popular in Britain since the sixteenth century. The oils found in bay leaves are mildly narcotic and have been used to soothe tension and hysteria. Bay is said to stimulate the appetite and its mellow flavour suits fish and grain dishes.

Chervil this herb resembles parsley but it has a more subtle flavour. Chervil can be mixed with other mild-flavoured herbs and used in fish, chicken and grain dishes. Sprigs of fresh chervil are also good in salads.

Chives this relative of the onion differs because the stalks and not the roots are used. Chives are easy to grow and will thrive in a pot in the kitchen or in a window bow. They are excellent chopped into salads or mixed with other herbs for savoury dishes.

Coriander both the stalks and the leaves of this herb are used in cooking and it has a slightly bitter, pungent flavour. Reputedly an aphrodisiac, coriander can be added to many savoury dishes and gives a subtle flavour to cooked fruits, muffins and mousses.

Dill named from an Anglo-Saxon word meaning 'to soothe', crushed dill seeds have been used to relieve flatulence and infant colic for centuries. Herbalists have also used dill to treat insomnia. The delicate, feathery leaves of this herb are traditional accompaniments to fish and egg dishes. It is delicious chopped into potato salads or added to coleslaws. Crushed dill seeds are not only soothing on the stomach but also excellent for flavouring salad dressings.

Garlic the most powerful member of the onion family, garlic has many unusual properties. Its first documented use as a medicine was in the Ebers papyrus over 3500 years ago when it was given to slaves working on the pyramids who enjoyed an exceptionally low rate of disease. In fact, the world's first recorded strike was when their garlic rations failed to appear. Garlic was also used extensively throughout early Chinese, Japanese and Roman dynasties as a food and medicine.

The garlic bulb grabs sulphurs from the soil as it grows and these are critical in its development. These sulphur compounds act as internal anti-bacterial and anti-fungal agents, and eating garlic is a good way of preventing stomach upsets when travelling. Taking garlic regularly in food or in capsules even deters mosquitos as the sulphur compounds are excreted through the skin and although we can't smell them, they deter the biting bugs. When garlic is chopped or crushed it releases a powerful substance called allicin. This affects the stickiness of blood platelets to keep the blood supply flowing smoothly and helps regulate blood fats such as cholesterol. Garlic is a useful ally in cases of high blood pressure and in the Mediterranean countries where it is used extensively there is a relatively low rate of heart disease.

Ginger native to Asia, ginger is an important part of Far Easten cookery. This spicy underground stem, or rhizome, may be bought fresh or dried but the freshly grated root has a better flavour. Ginger root is used extensively in Chinese herbal medicine and is one of the Four Official Capitals that form the basis of all their medications. Highly prized in the Middle Ages, a pound of ginger cost about the same as a sheep (in those days around 7p). Root ginger contains many essential oils and has been shown to thin the blood and lower cholesterol levels. Trials in Japan also report it to be an effective pain killer. Ginger can cure nausea and ginger tea made from a fresh infusion of the root is a safe and effective remedy for travel sickness or morning sickness. Grated ginger can be added to many sweet and savoury dishes. It works well with root vegetables, brassicas (such as cabbage), wholegrains and fish. It is also an excellent flavouring for melon and other fruits.

Horseradish this root comes from a relative of the nasturtium flower and is the richest plant source of sulphur. Used in herbal medicine to treat the liver and tone the system, horseradish has antibiotic qualities and can clear catarrh. Fresh horseradish may be minced and mixed with grated apple to accompany savoury dishes, but take care when handling as its vapour is highly irritating to the mucous membranes in the eyes and mouth. Used fresh it's extremely powerful in flavour, but slices of horseradish are less pungent than the grated root as fewer oils are released.

Marjoram this herb is one of our most popular and versatile herbs. Wild marjoram is also known as **oregano**, from Greek words meaning 'joy of the mountains'. Marjoram and oregano both contain high levels of thymol, a powerful antioxidant. Both herbs are widely used in Italian cooking and bring out the flavours of many foods, especially fish, cheese and wholegrain dishes.

Mint and spearmint were brought to Britain by the Romans and have been used extensively in British cooking. Mint sauce or mint jelly is the traditional accompaniment to roast lamb and their flavour complements richer foods. Traditionally used as a breath-freshener and digestive, the seventeenth-century herbalist Culpeper maintained mint was 'comfortable for the head and memory'. Peppermint tea is a refreshing after-dinner alternative to coffee that settles the stomach and may be served either hot or chilled.

Parsley this can be a difficult herb to grow, although it is said to flourish in households where the woman is in charge. Fresh parsley is rich in many vitamins and minerals and is a nutritious garnish or topping to almost every savoury dish. Herbalists prize parsley for its diuretic action and it is also used as a liver tonic. Sprigs of parsley make an interesting addition to salads and grain dishes, and parsley sauce works well with fish.

Rosemary the leaves of this herb contain a high concentration of natural oils which is why they are so highly scented. Rosemary is dedicated to friendship and traditionally sprigs were woven into Elizabethan wedding garlands. Herbalists associate rosemary with disorders of the head and it has been used to treat many problems from hair loss to migraine. Rosemary is also used to induce menstruation and it can raise blood pressure and boost the circulation. Rosemary works well with meat and oily fish dishes, and is a tasty addition to mixed herb blends.

Sage this small bushy herb has a strongly aromatic flavour and is said to be good for the brain and improve the memory. Sage may also stimulate the brain cortex and increase powers of concentration. It has also been recommended for longevity, possibly because of its high levels of natural oils. Sage tea is recommended by herbalists as a gargle for sore throats as it has a strongly antiseptic action. The pungent flavour of sage leaves complements heavier, fatty foods and its rich concentration of essential oils aids the digestion. Sage leaves are excellent with all types of cheese (they are used to make Sage Derby) and add flavour to blander dishes made with eggs and grains.

Tarragon used extensively in French cookery, tarragon leaves have a distinctive, spicy flavour. They are an important ingredient in many classical French recipes such as bearnaise and hollandaise sauces. Tarragon is closely related to wormwood, a bitter medicinal herb that has been used to induce abortions, so large amounts should be avoided by pregnant women. Tarragon gives an excellent flavour to many vegetable dishes and is useful for flavouring soups and sauces.

Thyme this is another herb that was brought to Britain by the Romans and it traditionally symbolises courage. One of our oldest herbalist, Culpeper refers to thyme as excellent for fighting infections. This is due to its high thymol content, thyme oil is a powerful antiseptic with many medicinal uses. Herbalists use thyme for chesty coughs and a few drops of the essential oil rubbed on the neck is a useful treatment for sore throats. In cooking, the strong flavour of thyme complements richer foods. In contrast, a few leaves will subtly flavour a salad dressing.

Spices

Herbs and spices are closely related and in some cases they come from the same plant. Generally, spices are recognised as being the seeds, berries, root or bark of plants that are native to tropical countries. All spices are highly scented and have been used in aromatic beauty preparations for thousands of years. One of the earliest Egyptian perfumes called *kyphi* contained several spices including cinnamon, juniper and cardamon. These aromatic spices are still used in many modern perfumes today.

When eaten, spices tend to be stimulating and antiseptic, for example, cinnamon is used in Indian medicine as a natural tonic for viral infections. Cloves are also traditionally used to boost the blood circulation and benefit the skin by bringing fresh oxygen supplies to its surface. Other spices, such as ginger and horse-radish, have powerful anti-infection properties and are especially useful for fending off coughs and colds.

Allspice from the dried fruit of a Jamaican evergreen tree. So-called because it tastes like a mixture of cinnamon, pepper and cloves. Used in tonics and digestives. An essential ingredient of Christmas pudding and hot mulled apple juice.

Caraway seeds these come from a relative of the carrot and have a distinctive flavour. The essential oil is used to make a liqueur and is said to improve digestion. The Greek physician Dioscorides prescribed caraway seeds for 'girls of pale face'. Used in German and Jewish cookery, caraway seeds are delicious with cabbage, cauliflower or added to rye bread and baked apples.

Cardamon pods from Sri Lanka, the pods should be cracked to release the seeds before using. Highly aromatic, a small amount of cardamon powder will go a long way and can be used to flavour both sweet and savoury dishes.

Cayenne pepper made from the dried fruit of the capsicum which belongs to the deadly nightshade family. The colour and flavour varies according to the variety of capsicum used. This type of pepper is hotter than black pepper and should be used with care.

Cinnamon made from the inner bark of a species of laurel tree that grows in Sri Lanka and India. Cinnamon sticks are made from bark scrapings and curl up while drying in the sun. Used by herbalists as a tonic, small doses can improve the blood circulation. For the best flavour, buy cinnamon in sticks and grind as needed. Delicious added to many fruit dishes, especially stewed apple, melon and pear compotes. Cinnamon also blends well with other spices such as allspice and cloves.

Cloves these tiny dried buds come from an evergreen tree in Indonesia. Clove oil is a powerful local anaesthetic and can be bought in bottles from chemists for the relief of toothache (alternatively, chew a clove). Cloves should be used sparingly but are excellent to flavour fruit, bread sauce, poultry and game.

Cumin these dried seeds were used extensively in Roman times and a recipe from an early gourmet called Apicius in AD 300 quotes cumin and parsley to flavour shellfish. Cumin seeds come from the Mediterranean and are popular in Middle Eastern cookery. They have a pungent, bitter flavour and a distinctive aroma. Useful for stimulating the appetite and soothing the digestion, cumin works best with savoury dishes and is a traditional ingredient of Moroccan cookery.

Nutmeg these are the dried seeds from an evergreen tree that grows in the Molucca Islands in Indonesia. The seeds are covered in a stiff red web which is removed and sold separately as mace. Nutmegs are best bought whole and grated as required to preserve their flavour. Popular in British cooking for centuries, women sometimes wore a silver nutmeg box and grater on a cord around their waist. Freshly grated mace or nutmeg is traditionally used to flavour fish, sauces, custards and egg dishes. It is also excellent with rice pudding and stewed fruits. However, both mace and nutmeg contain *myristicin*, which is toxic in large doses, so use sparingly, especially in recipes for children.

Paprika made from the dried fruit of a mild red capsicum mainly grown in Spain. Its flavour is milder than other types of pepper and it is good for adding colour and flavour to pulse and grain dishes.

Pepper peppercorns are the dried, unripened fruit of an Indian vine and can be bought whole or pre-ground. Several varieties are available, including black pepper from dried, unripe green peppercorns and white pepper made from ripe red peppercorns. Both have more flavour when freshly ground from a pepper mill. Pepper is useful to bring out the flavour in many savoury foods and those wishing to cut down on their salt intake can season foods with freshly ground black pepper and lemon juice.

Poppy seeds poppies became notorious after the discovery of opium and its narcotic derivatives. However, poppy seeds used for cooking come from a different variety of the flower and do not contain morphine or codeine. Rich in natural oils, poppy seeds have been eaten since Roman times and are an important part of Jewish cookery. Poppy seeds can be added to breads, biscuits, rice and grain dishes.

Saffron these vivid yellow strands come from the saffron crocus and have been popular in recipes for centuries. Originally brought to Britain during the reign of Edward III in 1460, saffron was cultivated in the South of England and gave the name to Saffron Walden in Essex and Saffron Hill in central London. It is an expensive spice as around 50,000 stamens from the crocus flower are needed to produce each pound of saffron, each one being picked by hand. Saffron strands give savoury dishes a mildly aromatic flavour but are mainly used to dye foods such as bread and rice a vivid shade of yellow.

Turmeric a rhizome or underground stem from the ginger family, turmeric is the basic ingredient of curry powder. It is used in herbal medicine as a stimulant and can also be used in cooking as a vivid yellow dye.

Vanilla the long dark pods from this climbing orchid plant are dried and used mainly to scent and flavour sweet dishes such as custards and mousses. Although the dried pods are expensive, they can be rinsed and re-used many times and taste a good deal better than synthetic vanilla essence.

RECIPES

Beautiful Breakfasts

Breakfast is a meal not to be missed as it gives you energy for the day ahead. Begin the day as you mean to go on and treat yourself to a healthy start.

SUPER SEED SHAKE

This fast milk shake is full of calcium and iron. Extra supplies of sunflower and sesame seeds may be ground and stored in the fridge to save preparation time. The shake tastes best when chilled, so keep your cartons of soya milk or apple juice in the fridge beforehand.

SERVES 2

1 level tablespoon sunflower seeds
1 level tablespoon sesame seeds
300 ml (½ pint) skimmed milk, soya milk or
 apple juice
1 teaspoon crude blackstrap molasses
1 ripe banana, peeled (optional)

Finely grind the sunflower and sesame seeds in a coffee mill. Blend the ground seeds, milk or apple juice, molasses and banana (if using) together.

BUCKWHEAT PANCAKES

A Sunday breakfast family treat, try these tasty pancakes spread with a little real maple syrup and lemon juice, or roll them round a large spoonful of low-fat fromage frais. For a savoury filling, try stir-fried vegetable strips sprinkled with tamari sauce.

SERVES 6/MAKES ABOUT 20 PANCAKES

100 g (4 oz) buckwheat flour
100 g (4 oz) brown rice flour
2 free-range eggs (size 3), lightly beaten
600 ml (1 pint) soya milk
2 tablespoons sesame or cold-pressed olive oil for frying

Pre-heat the oven to 120°C, 250°F (gas mark ½). Sift the flours together into a basin and make a well in the centre. Add the beaten egg and gradually beat in the soya milk incorporating all the flour to make a smooth batter. Leave the batter to stand for 30 minutes.

To cook the pancakes, stir the batter, then heat a little oil in a frying pan. Quickly pour in a tablespoonful of batter to coat the base of the pan thinly. Cook the pancake until light brown underneath, then flip it over with a palette knife or fish slice and cook the other side. Slide the pancake on to a warmed heatproof dish, roll it up and place in the oven to keep warm. Continue making the remaining pancakes in the same way.

HOT BULGAR BREAKFAST

This delicious, nutritious hot cereal is a perfect winter-warmer for cold, dark days. Serve plain or with a little additional milk or soya milk.

SERVES 4

1 tablespoon unrefined oil (e.g. virgin olive oil)
150 g (5 oz) bulgar wheat (cracked wheat)
100 g (4 oz) sesame seeds
100 g (4 oz) wheatgerm
600 ml (1 pint) water
25 g (1 oz) dried apricots, finely chopped
25 g (1 oz) raisins or currants
25 g (1 oz) chopped hazelnuts or almonds

Gently heat the oil in a large saucepan, add the bulgar wheat, sesame seeds and wheatgerm, and lightly sauté until slightly browned. Add the water and stir in the dried fruits. Cover and simmer for about 25 minutes or until the bulgar is fluffy and the water has been absorbed. Add nuts to taste and serve immediately.

BIRCHER MUESLI

This recipe is based on the original muesli invented by Dr Bircher-Benner for patients at his famous natural health clinic in Switzerland. To save time in the mornings, the oats may be soaked overnight, leaving only the fruit and hazelnuts to be added at breakfast. Dr Bircher-Benner believed that the entire apple should be used – pips and all!

SERVES 2

4 tablespoons rolled oats
2 tablespoons low-fat, live yoghurt
6 tablespoons cold water
½ teaspoon grated lemon rind
225 g (8 oz) freshly grated (unpeeled) apple
or
450 g (1 lb) seasonal soft fruits
2 tablespoons chopped hazelnuts

Put the oats, yoghurt, water and lemon rind into a large bowl and stir until creamy. Leave in the fridge overnight if preferred. Add the fruit and serve sprinkled with the chopped hazelnuts.

Starters And Snacks

CREAM OF CELERY SOUP

This soup should ideally be served smooth but it can also be prepared leaving out the puréeing stage.

SERVES 4–6

1 tablespoon sesame oil
2 onions, peeled and finely chopped
10 stalks celery, chopped
40 g (1½ oz) oat flakes
1.25 litres (2¼ pints) water
1 teaspoon freshly chopped thyme or dill

Heat the sesame oil in a saucepan and sauté the onions until transparent. Add the chopped celery and sauté for another few minutes. Stir in the oat flakes and gently cook for about 5 minutes until they are well-coated with the sesame oil and moistened. Slowly stir in the water, cover and simmer over a low heat for 30–40 minutes. Purée the soup in a food processor until smooth. Serve sprinkled with the fresh herbs.

BARLEY AND VEGETABLE SOUP

A hearty, nourishing soup that satisfies the hungriest of stomachs. This recipe works particularly well with root vegetables, such as carrot, parsnip and swede.

SERVES 4

3 tablespoons cold-pressed olive oil
2 onions, peeled and chopped
450 g (1 lb) any vegetable, chopped, diced or shredded
75 g (3 oz) pot barley
½ teaspoon freshly grated root ginger
1.2 litres (2 pints) vegetable stock
Freshly ground black pepper

In a large saucepan, heat the oil and lightly sauté the onions and the other vegetable of your choice. Stir in the pot barley, root ginger, stock and season with the freshly ground black pepper. Cover and simmer over a low heat for 2 hours or until the barley is soft.

BUCKWHEAT NOODLE SOUP

A satisfying soup made with nourishing noodles and kombu seaweed (see page 136).

SERVES 2–3

2.75 litres (5 pints) water plus 350 ml (12 fl oz) water
225 g (8 oz) buckwheat noodles
8 spring onions, trimmed and finely chopped
1 tablespoon cold-pressed olive oil
750 ml (1¼ pints) water
3-inch piece kombu seaweed
3 tablespoons tamari sauce

Bring the 2.75 litres (5 pints) of water to the boil in a large saucepan. Add the buckwheat noodles and bring the water back to the boil, then add 120 ml (4 fl oz) cold water. Repeat the process of bringing the water back to the boil and adding the cold water three times all told.

Take the saucepan off the heat, cover and leave for 10 minutes. Drain and rinse the noodles in cold water and set aside.

To make the soup: heat the oil in a saucepan and sauté the spring onions for a few minutes. Add the 750 ml (1¼ pints) water and the kombu seaweed, and bring to the boil. Cover and simmer for 15 minutes. Remove the kombu seaweed and set on one side. Stir the tamari sauce into the soup and bring back to the boil. Meanwhile re-heat the noodles by pouring boiling water over them. Drain and put the noodles into warmed bowls with the kombu seaweed, and pour over the soup.

ONION SOUP

This simple soup is easy to prepare. If you prefer to omit the grated cheese it becomes a recipe very low in calories too. If adding the cheese, however, choose a full-flavoured variety such as mature Cheddar, Gruyère or Emmenthal. You can either make the carrot juice in an electric juicer, or buy it in bottles or cartons from most supermarkets.

SERVES 2

2 tablespoons cold-pressed olive oil
4 onions, peeled and finely sliced
600 ml (1 pint) vegetable stock, carrot juice or mixed
    vegetable juice
A dash of Worcestershire sauce
Pinch of freshly ground black pepper
1 bay leaf
2 tablespoons grated cheese (optional)

Heat the oil in a large saucepan and fry the onions until transparent and soft. Add the stock or juice, the Worcestershire sauce, black pepper and bay leaf, cover the pan and simmer for at least 20 minutes to allow the full flavour to develop. Remove the bay leaf and serve sprinkled with grated cheese (optional).

MUSHROOM PATE

This is very useful for packed lunches or spread on rice cakes as a starter or snack. I find that the larger varieties of mushrooms have more flavour.

SERVES 4–6

225 g (8 oz) mushrooms, roughly chopped
1 clove garlic, peeled and crushed
1 tablespoon cold-pressed olive oil
2 tablespoons white wine
50 g (2 oz) almonds or hazelnuts
2 tablespoons very low-fat fromage frais

For the garnish
Slivers of red and yellow pepper

Heat the oil in a large frying pan and briefly fry the mushrooms and garlic before adding the white wine. Simmer until the mushrooms are cooked and the cooking liquid has been absorbed. Place the mixture in a food processor with the almonds or hazelnuts and blend into a coarse paste. Fold in the fromage frais and chill before serving, garnished with thin slices of red and yellow pepper.

HUMUS

This is also a delicious filling for sandwiches or baked potatoes, or is very tasty on rye crackers or rice cakes.

SERVES 2–4

50 g (2 oz) cooked chick peas (see page 74)
Juice of 1 lemon
2 cloves garlic, peeled and crushed
1 tablespoon cold-pressed olive oil
1 tablespoon tahini
50 ml (2 fl oz) water (optional)

For the garnish
1 tablespoon freshly chopped parsley
1 tablespoon pine kernels

If using a food processor, place all the ingredients in the bowl and blend until smooth. Alternatively, place all the ingredients into a large mixing bowl and pound with a potato masher, if necessary adding a little water to make the mixture smooth. Serve garnished with parsley and pine nuts.

Sensational Salads And Vegetables

WARM GOAT'S CHEESE SALAD

Goat's cheese is more easily digested than cheese made from cow's milk as its fat and protein molecules are much smaller. This is because it is intended to feed a baby goat which, unlike a calf, is similar in size to a human baby.

SERVES 4

175 g (6 oz) goat's cheese
1 tablespoon cold-pressed olive oil
2 tablespoons Fine French dressing (see page 180)
16 mixed salad leaves
50 g (2 oz) sunflower seeds

Pre-heat the grill or the oven to 180°C, 350°F (gas mark 4).

Slice the goat's cheese into four thick slices. Brush a baking tray with the olive oil and place the cheese slices on it. Heat in the oven or under a medium grill until melted and lightly browned. Meanwhile, toss the salad leaves in the French dressing and arrange on four small plates. Place one slice of goat's cheese in the centre. Sprinkle with sunflower seeds and serve immediately.

SPINACH WITH YOGHURT DRESSING

This is delicious served with Tofu and Onion Flan (page 186) or Millet croquettes (page 192).

SERVES 4

150 ml (¼ pint) natural low-fat, live yoghurt
1 tablespoon olive oil
1 tablespoon lemon juice or cider vinegar
1 teaspoon finely chopped onion
1 tablespoon chopped fresh mint
1 clove garlic, peeled and split in two
225 g (8 oz) fresh, young spinach leaves

For the garnish
A few sprigs of fresh mint
2 radishes, thinly sliced

Combine the yoghurt, olive oil, lemon juice or cider vinegar, onion and mint to make the dressing. Place the garlic pieces in the dressing or, for a stronger garlic flavour, squeeze the juice from the clove into the dressing. Toss the spinach leaves in the dressing and chill for one hour.

Garnish with the mint leaves and radish slices before serving.

VITAMIN SALAD

This salad can be adapted to include any of your favourite vegetables. All the vegetables should be raw. Vitamin salad is especially good served with Orange and Tamari Dressing (see page 182) or use the Fine French dressing (see page 180).

50 g (2 oz) Brussels sprouts, grated
50 g (2 oz) parsnip, peeled and grated
50 g (2 oz) swede, peeled and grated
50 g (2 oz) raw beetroot, grated
50 g (2 oz) radishes, trimmed and thinly sliced
50 g (2 oz) olives, finely diced
50 g (2 oz) cabbage, shredded
50 g (2 oz) celery, chopped
1 small onion, peeled and finely chopped
50 g (2 oz) watercress or mustard and cress
Salad dressing of your choice

Mix all the ingredients together in a large bowl and stir in your favourite dressing.

TABBOULEH

SERVES 6

175 g (6 oz) bulgar wheat (cracked wheat)
4 spring onions, trimmed and finely chopped
1 medium-sized cucumber, finely chopped
4 tablespoons freshly chopped parsley
1–2 tablespoons freshly chopped mint
1–2 tablespoons freshly chopped basil
Freshly squeezed juice of 1 lemon
4 tablespoons cold-pressed olive or unrefined hazelnut oil

For the garnish
6 slivers red pepper or pimento
6 chopped black olives

Rinse the bulgar wheat thoroughly before soaking it in cold water for at least an hour. Drain well.

Add the finely chopped spring onions, cucumber and herbs to the lemon juice and oil and mix together well. Pour the mixture over the bulgar wheat and stir thoroughly. Serve garnished with slivers of red pepper or pimento and chopped black olives.

SUNSHINE SALAD

This salad makes an attractive starter or light lunch dish. You can adapt the recipe according to the salad leaves and fresh herbs available. Sun-dried tomatoes (in bottles) are available from larger delicatessens and Italian food shops.

SERVES 6

For the dressing
150 ml (¼ pint) cold-pressed olive oil
25 ml (1 fl oz) fresh lime juice
2 teaspoons French mustard
Freshly ground black pepper

For the salad
4 large carrots, scrubbed and grated
225 g (8 oz) mixed salad leaves, such as spinach, radiccio, frisee, oakleaf and batavia lettuces, endive and lamb's lettuce
50 g (2 oz) mixed herb leaves, such as chervil, basil and roquette
50 g (2 oz) sun-dried tomatoes, finely chopped
50 g (2 oz) hazelnuts, almonds or pecans, finely chopped

Mix together the dressing ingredients. Pour half the dressing over the grated carrots.

Put the carrots in the centre of a large, flat serving platter. Arrange the mixed salad and herb leaves round the outside. Sprinkle with the chopped, sun-dried tomatoes and nuts. Pour on the remaining salad dressing and serve immediately.

Delicious Dressings

Dressings are the fastest ways to liven up raw vegetables and salad combinations. The thicker ones based on yoghurt can also be used as dips for raw vegetables.

FINE FRENCH DRESSING

Stored tightly sealed in the fridge this dressing will keep for up to a week.

MAKES 300 ML (½ PINT)

175 ml (6 fl oz) unrefined sunflower or safflower oil
120 ml (4 fl oz) lemon juice
Freshly ground black pepper
½ teaspoon mustard
¼ teaspoon freshly grated root ginger
1–2 large cloves garlic, peeled and crushed

Put all the ingredients in a screw-top jar, replace the lid and shake vigorously to mix well.

CUCUMBER DRESSING

A delicious, refreshing dressing that also works well on baked potatoes and sliced avocados.

SERVES 2–4

150 g (5 oz) cucumber
150 g (5 oz) natural low-fat, live yoghurt
1 tablespoon cider vinegar
1 sprig of dill
½ teaspoon dried dill seeds

Blend all the ingredients together in a food processor until the dressing is smooth and creamy.

YOGHURT AND CHIVE DRESSING

SERVES 2–4

150 ml (¼ pint) natural low-fat, live yoghurt
1 tablespoon cold-pressed olive oil
1 tablespoon lemon juice
1 teaspoon Dijon mustard
2 tablespoons chopped chives
1 clove garlic, peeled and crushed
Freshly ground black pepper

In a large bowl, mix all the ingredients together, adding black pepper to season, and stir vigorously. Alternatively, place the ingredients in a large, screw-top jar, replace the lid and shake well.

ORANGE AND TAMARI DRESSING

This is very good with green-leafed vegetables such as raw spinach or salad leaves. It is also a useful dressing for those who dislike using vinegar.

SERVES 2–4

150 ml (¼ pint) freshly squeezed orange juice
1 teaspoon grated orange peel
2 tablespoons tamari sauce
1 teaspoon finely chopped fresh root ginger
3 tablespoons cold-pressed olive oil
1 clove garlic, peeled and crushed

In a large bowl, mix all the ingredients together and stir well before using. Alternatively, place the ingredients into a large, screw-top jar, replace the lid and shake well.

Magnificent Main Meals

This section includes ideas for filling family meals, as well as lighter lunch dishes.

HOME-MADE HERB SAUSAGES

At last – no need to worry about the additives! These brilliant bangers can be made with either lamb or pork. The pork sausages must be cooked all the way through, but the lamb sausages may be left slightly pink inside.

EACH ALTERNATIVE MAKES 8–10 SAUSAGES

Cold-pressed olive oil, for frying (optional)
450 g (1 lb) lean lamb or pork, diced
1 small onion, peeled and roughly chopped
1 teaspoon French mustard
1 free-range egg, size 3
25 g (1 oz) buckwheat flour or barley flour for coating

For the lamb sausages
4 large sprigs of fresh mint or basil, roughly chopped

For the pork sausages
4 large sprigs of fresh sage, roughly chopped

Mix all the ingredients in a food processor until the mixture resembles sausage meat (this may take a few minutes). Divide the mixture into eight portions and, with floured hands, roll each into a sausage shape. The bangers can either be shallow fried in a little olive oil or cooked under a pre-heated grill.

CABBAGE PARCELS

SERVES 6

100 g (4 oz) millet
450 ml (15 fl oz) vegetable or chicken stock
1 savoy cabbage
1 tablespoon cold-pressed olive oil
2 red onions, peeled and chopped
4 spring onions, sliced into rings
8 stems of fresh coriander
2 cloves garlic, peeled and crushed
3 carrots, chopped
2 leeks, chopped
4 tomatoes, chopped
100 g (4 oz) okra, chopped
Juice of 1 lime
Freshly ground black pepper
2 tablespoons water or stock

Pre-heat the oven to 180°C, 350°F (gas mark 4).

Place the millet and stock in a saucepan, bring to the boil, cover and simmer for about 20 minutes or until the millet is soft.

Separate the cabbage into whole leaves and blanch them in boiling water for 30 seconds. Set aside to drain on kitchen paper.

Chop the stems of the coriander. Chop the leaves and set on one side. Heat the oil and gently fry the onion, coriander stems and garlic until the onion is transparent. Add the chopped carrots and leeks and continue to cook for another minute. Add the tomatoes, okra, the chopped coriander leaves and stir in the cooked millet. Add the lime juice, and freshly ground black pepper to season.

Place a dessertspoonful of the millet mixture on a cabbage leaf and roll up, folding in the sides as you go. Repeat until all the cabbage leaves have been filled. Place in an ovenproof dish, spoon over 2 tablespoons of water or stock, cover and bake for 20 minutes.

MAJESTIC MINCE

This hearty and filling recipe replaces the saturated fat content of the minced meat with healthier vegetable oils. Serve with baked potatoes, brown rice or wholewheat pasta shells.

SERVES 3–4

225 g (8 oz) lean minced beef or lamb (preferably organically reared)
3 tablespoons cold-pressed olive oil or unrefined sunflower oil
2 leeks, thinly sliced
¼ small cabbage, chopped
4 carrots, thinly sliced
1 teaspoon freshly chopped rosemary
1 teaspoon freshly chopped oregano
450 g (1 lb) tomatoes, chopped or
400 g (1 × 14 oz) tin chopped tomatoes
Freshly ground black pepper

Put the mince in a microwave oven, or in a heavy-based saucepan on top of the stove, and heat until cooked. Pour all the meat juices and fat into a basin, and set on one side to go cold. Skim off the fat and pour only the juices back into the meat.

Gently heat the olive or sunflower oil in a saucepan over a low heat and add the leeks, cabbage and carrots. Cover and simmer for 5 minutes or until the vegetables are soft. Add the mince with the juices, the rosemary, oregano, tomatoes, and freshly ground black pepper to season. Simmer for a further 5 minutes to allow the full flavour to develop.

TOFU AND ONION FLAN

A delicious dairy and gluten-free flan made with buckwheat pastry. Serve hot with Baked Beetroot (see page 196) and steamed broccoli.

SERVES 4

For the pastry
100 g (4 oz) buckwheat flour
25 g (1 oz) poppy seeds
2 tablespoons unrefined walnut or hazelnut oil
50 ml (2 fl oz) ice-cold water

For the filling
1 teaspoon cold-pressed olive oil for frying
225 g (8 oz) red onions, peeled and finely sliced
225 g (8 oz) white onions, peeled and finely sliced
225 g (8 oz) firm silken tofu
150 ml (¼ pint) soya milk
2 teaspoons mustard
Freshly ground black pepper
2 free-range eggs, size 3

Pre-heat the oven to 200°C, 400°F (gas mark 6); then 160°C, 325°F (gas mark 3).

Mix the flour and poppy seeds in a food processor, and slowly dribble in the oil. Add only enough of the water to enable the dough to form a ball round the blade. Put the dough in a bowl, cover with a cloth and place in the fridge for 30 minutes.

Heat the olive oil and fry the onions until transparent. Place the tofu in the food processor and blend until smooth and the consistency of double cream. Add the other ingredients and blend again.

Roll out the pastry and use to line a 20 cm (8 inch) flan dish. Bake blind for 10 minutes. Reduce the oven temperature. Arrange the onions in the pastry case and pour over the tofu mixture. Bake for 45 minutes or until set and turning golden brown.

FAST FISH RISOTTO

This risotto is a good way to use up pre-cooked rice, and the frozen peas are an excellent source of fibre and protein. Tinned fish such as tuna or salmon may be substituted for the fresh oily fish.

SERVES 2

100 g (4 oz) fresh oily fish (e.g. mackerel or herring)
1 onion, peeled and finely chopped
1 tablespoon cold-pressed olive oil
6 heaped tablespoons cooked brown rice
150 g (5 oz) frozen peas
1 tablespoon freshly chopped basil or parsley

Cook the fish under a hot grill for about 5 minutes, turning it once. Allow to cool slightly, then flake the fish flesh into large pieces.

Heat the oil in a large frying pan and lightly fry the onion. Add the fish, the rice and peas. Stir continuously to prevent the mixture sticking to the sides of the saucepan while heating through for about 3 minutes to cook the peas.

Garnish with the chopped basil or parsley before serving.

BUCKWHEAT BONANZA

This buckwheat feast works well with the stronger flavours of wild mushrooms such as the shiitake or oyster varieties. If you have the time, fresh artichoke hearts are the tastiest, otherwise, tinned artichoke hearts can be used.

SERVES 2

50 g (2 oz) roasted buckwheat (kasha)
50 g (2 oz) buckwheat
450 ml (¾ pint) water
100 g (4 oz) artichoke hearts
1 tablespoon cold-pressed olive oil
100 g (4 oz) button or wild mushrooms, roughly chopped
4 spring onions, chopped
1 teaspoon dried sage and parsley or 2 teaspoons chopped
    fresh sage and parsley
1 teaspoon tamari sauce
Freshly ground black pepper
25 g (1 oz) pecan nuts (optional)

Rinse the buckwheats in a sieve under a running tap. Bring the water to the boil, add the buckwheats, cover and simmer for 15 minutes or until soft.

Meanwhile, if using fresh artichokes, trim and cook them in minimal water or in a steamer. When soft, remove the leaves and trim away the toughened fibres to reveal the soft hearts. If using tinned artichoke hearts these will be pre-cooked. Roughly chop the artichokes.

In a large frying pan heat the oil and gently soften the mushrooms and spring onions. Drain and add the buckwheat, chopped artichokes and herbs, and stir well. Add the tamari sauce, and freshly ground black pepper to season. Serve sprinkled with pecan nuts, if using.

REALLY EASY ROAST CHICKEN

It's not much more fiddly to include the Apricot Stuffing (see below), but I'll leave the choice to you.

1 fresh free-range chicken
1 tablespoon cold-pressed olive oil
2 tablespoons chopped, fresh mixed herbs
or 1 tablespoon dried mixed herbs
Freshly ground black pepper
1 recipe quantity Apricot Stuffing (see below)

Pre-heat the oven to 200°C, 400°F (gas mark 6).

Place the chicken in a roasting tray. Brush with the olive oil and sprinkle with herbs and freshly ground black pepper. Roast in the oven for 20 minutes per lb plus 10–20 minutes extra. Baste the chicken from time to time. To test if it's cooked insert a skewer into the thickest part of the thigh. The juices should run clear. Allow the chicken to stand in a warm place for 10 minutes before carving.

APRICOT STUFFING

To stuff one 1.75 kg (4 lb) chicken

175 g (6 oz) dried apricots, chopped
175 g (6 oz) fresh, wholewheat breadcrumbs
½ teaspoon lemon juice
4 tablespoons cold-pressed olive oil
Freshly ground black pepper

Soak the chopped apricots in cold water for about 30 minutes or until plump and soft. Stir into the breadcrumbs. Add the lemon juice, olive oil and freshly ground black pepper to season. Work some of the stuffing firmly over the breast and secure the neck flap to keep the stuffing in place. Spoon the remaining stuffing inside the cavity of the chicken.

RED CABBAGE WITH APPLE

This delicious side dish is cooked like a stir-fry, so you need to watch it if cooking it on top of the stove. Alternatively, this dish can also be baked in an ovenproof dish for 15 minutes at 180°C, 350°F (gas mark 4). Its ruby red colour brightens a pale plate of cooked grains and it complements chicken and fish dishes well.

SERVES 4

1 tablespoon cold-pressed olive oil
225 g (8 oz) red cabbage, shredded
2 eating apples, cored and grated (preferably unpeeled)
1 teaspoon clear honey
1 teaspoon cider vinegar
Freshly ground black pepper

Heat the oil in a large pan and briefly sauté the cabbage before adding the apples. Then add the honey, vinegar and freshly ground black pepper to season. Cover and cook gently for 5 minutes.

The Gorgeous Gourmet

If the very thought of entertaining throws your resolve for healthy eating out of the window, read on. Many of the most exotic foods are also the best for us. What could be more lavish than half a juicy cantaloupe melon filled with strawberries? And yet this simple starter is the ultimate in eating yourself beautiful. Or how about skewers of seafood served with saffron rice, or artichokes drizzled with hazelnut oil? And for dessert it's hard to beat a tropical fruit salad served with slivers of almonds. The ideas are so easy – fresh, wholesome food prepared and presented in an inspiring way.

TAPENADE

This rich olive paste comes from Provence and can be used to coat chicken breasts, fish fillets or cubes of tofu. Or simply serve it hot with a mixture of rices and green beans or as an appetiser spread on small chunks of rye bread. Tapenade does not need any cooking.

MAKES 175 G (6 OZ)

100 g (4 oz) pitted black olives, chopped
2 tablespoons capers, rinsed in milk to remove excess salt
2 cloves garlic, peeled and crushed
3 tablespoons extra virgin olive or hazelnut oil
Freshly ground black pepper
Chopped fresh oregano or basil or thyme to taste

If using the tapenade to coat chicken, fish or tofu, pre-heat the oven to 180°C, 350°F (gas mark 4).

Blend all the ingredients together in a food processor or pass them through a sieve to form a smooth paste. To coat the chicken, fish or tofu chunks, simply spread with tapenade mixture and bake in the oven for 15 –20 minutes.

MILLET CROQUETTES

Both children and adults love these. Serve them warm with a tomato sauce (made simply by cooking and puréeing fresh tomatoes). Cooked brown rice may be substituted for the millet.

MAKES 18

450 g (1 lb) cooked millet
1 onion, peeled and finely chopped
100 g (4 oz) green vegetables (e.g. broccoli or beans or
    courgettes), chopped
2 tablespoons tamari sauce
50 g (2 oz) wholewheat plain flour
150 ml (¼ pint) water or vegetable stock (optional)
1 teaspoon cold-pressed olive oil to grease the baking sheet

Pre-heat the oven to 200°C, 400°F (gas mark 6).

Mix all the ingredients except the water or stock together in a large bowl and knead for 5–10 minutes. If the dough seems too stiff, add a little water or vegetable stock to soften it (if it is a little loose, add additional flour). Roll the mixture into small balls and press flat. Lay the croquettes on a lightly oiled baking sheet and bake for 20 minutes.

FIVE VEGETABLE TERRINE

This multi-coloured terrine may be served hot or cold. For an attractive starter, slice and serve it in the centre of a plate of freshly squeezed (or bottled) tomato juice.

SERVES 6–8

450 g (1 lb) carrots, cubed
225 g (8 oz) celeriac, peeled and cubed
350 g (12 oz) fresh spinach
350 g (12 oz) broccoli, broken into florets
225 g (8 oz) leeks, white part only, sliced
Freshly ground black pepper
Juice of 1 orange
6 free-range eggs, size 3

Pre-heat the oven to 200°C, 400°F (gas mark 6).

Cook the carrots and celeriac in boiling water in separate saucepans until tender. Cook the spinach in a little water for about 5–6 minutes. Blanch the broccoli and leeks in boiling water, separately, for 1–2 minutes. Drain all the vegetables well.

In a food processor, blend the leek and celeriac with a pinch of black pepper and two eggs until puréed to a coarse texture. Repeat, using the broccoli, spinach and two of the eggs. Finally, repeat the process with the carrot, adding the orange juice and two remaining eggs.

Line a 1 kg (2 lb) loaf tin with lightly oiled baking parchment or greaseproof paper. Spread the green spinach and broccoli mixture over the bottom and follow with a cream-coloured layer of leek and celeriac. Finally, top with a layer of carrot and orange purée. Place the loaf tin inside a large roasting tin filled with about 1 cm (½ inch) of hot water. Bake for about 1 hour or until set. Turn out on a serving dish, allow to cool slightly then peel off the baking parchment before slicing the terrine.

SEAFOOD SPEARS

Choose fish with a firm flesh, such as cod, tuna or salmon, so that it will thread easily on to skewers. Serve on a bed of mixed brown and wild rices.

SERVES 4

For the marinade
4 tablespoons unrefined sunflower or safflower oil
Juice of 1 lemon
1 tablespoon tamari sauce
1 tablespoon fresh chopped parsley
Freshly ground black pepper

For the spears
8 shallots, peeled or 2 large onions, peeled and quartered
750 g (1½ lb) fresh or frozen fish
8 scallops or large prawns
½ red and ½ green pepper, de-seeded and cubed
2 courgettes, thickly sliced

For the garnish
1 tablespoon chopped fresh parsley

Combine the ingredients for the marinade. Blanch the shallots or onions for 1 minute in boiling water.

Cut the fish into chunks and thread together with the scallops or prawns, shallots or onions, peppers and courgettes on to wooden or metal skewers. Brush with the marinade and place under a medium heat grill and cook for about 5 minutes (depending upon the fish). Turn the kebabs twice, brushing them with marinade as they cook. Garnish with chopped parsley before serving.

ASPARAGUS AND MUSHROOM RISOTTO

To make this tasty light supper dish even more exotic add a pinch of saffron to the cooking liquid to turn the rice yellow. Also, try mixing two types of rice (e.g. brown basmati and brown Italian rice) for added variety.

SERVES 2 AS A MAIN DISH OR 4 AS A STARTER

100 g (4 oz) brown rice (mixed if possible), well rinsed
475 ml (16 fl oz) water
1 large onion, peeled and finely chopped
Few strands of saffron (optional)
100 g (4 oz) fresh asparagus, trimmed
2 teaspoons cold-pressed olive oil
100 g (4 oz) mushrooms, finely chopped
2 tablespoons chopped fresh parsley
Freshly ground black pepper
Juice of ½ lemon

Gently heat a heavy-based saucepan on top of the stove, add the rice and stir with a wooden spatula for 1 minute until lightly toasted. Add the water, onion and saffron, if using. Bring to the boil, cover and simmer for 20 minutes.

Meanwhile, chop the asparagus into short lengths, reserving the tips for garnish. After the 20 minutes cooking time add the lengths of asparagus and simmer for another 10–15 minutes until the rice is soft.

In a separate pan, gently heat the olive oil and lightly sauté the asparagus tips. Remove from the pan and drain on kitchen paper. Stir the chopped mushrooms and parsley into the cooked rice mixture. Season with black pepper, stir in the lemon juice and serve garnished with the asparagus tips.

PRAWN KEBABS WITH HERB DRESSING

SERVES 2

For the kebabs
12 king-sized prawns
8 button mushrooms
1 medium courgette, sliced

For the herb dressing
4 tablespoons cold-pressed olive or unrefined sunflower oil
1 clove garlic, peeled and crushed
Juice of 1 lemon
1 sprig each of basil, parsley and tarragon, finely chopped

Thread the prawns, button mushrooms and sliced courgette on to wooden or metal skewers and place in a shallow dish. Mix the ingredients for the herb dressing together thoroughly and pour over the threaded skewers. Cover and leave to marinate for 30 minutes, turning them occasionally.

Place under a medium heat grill and cook for about 3 minutes, basting and turning the kebabs as they cook.

BAKED BEETROOT

Delicious hot or cold, serve plain or with a spoonful of yoghurt.

SERVES 4

4 whole, raw beetroot

Pre-heat the oven to 160°C, 325°F (gas mark 3).

Scrub the beetroot clean. Trim, leaving the roots and one inch of the stems intact on each beet. Put the beetroot on a baking sheet and bake for ½–1 hour (depending upon size) until tender when pierced with a skewer. Peel away the skin and serve sliced.

Superb Sauces

A tasty sauce is one of the simplest and best ways to liven up plainly cooked wholegrains and pulses. These recipes contain many unusual ingredients such as tahini, which is made from crushed sesame seeds, and miso which comes from soya beans. Several of the recipes are either dairy- or gluten-free and are particularly useful for those on restricted diets.

CREAMY MUSTARD SAUCE

To use on fresh fish (e.g. herrings or salmon), baked chicken breasts or lean lamb chops.

SERVES 2

3 tablespoons fat-free fromage frais
2 teaspoons mild French mustard
A little chopped tarragon, fresh or dried
Freshly ground black pepper

Mix all the ingredients together in a small saucepan, adding freshly ground black pepper to season. Heat gently, stirring, taking care not to let the mixture boil. Serve immediately.

BÉCHAMEL SAUCE

An unusual dairy and gluten-free alternative to white sauce.

SERVES 2

½ teaspoon cold-pressed olive or sesame oil
1 small onion, peeled and chopped
1 spring onion, trimmed and sliced
1 tablespoon rice flour
300 ml (½ pint) water
½ tablespoon tahini

Heat the oil and sauté the onion and spring onion for a few minutes. Sprinkle in the flour, stirring constantly. Gradually add the water and slowly bring to the boil. Boil for a few minutes to cook the flour and stir in the tahini. Simmer gently for 15 minutes, half covered with a lid.

LYONNAISE SAUCE

This goes well with white fish, pork, tofu and Quorn.

SERVES 2

1 teaspoon cold-pressed olive oil
1 small onion, peeled and minced or grated
1 tablespoon apple juice
½ recipe quantity Béchamel sauce (see above)

Heat the oil and sauté the onion for a few minutes. Add the apple juice, cover and cook gently until the onion has softened. Mix with the béchamel sauce and heat through, if necessary.

MISO SAUCE

Miso is made from fermented soya beans and is sold in health food shops. It is an important ingredient in macrobiotic cooking and has a deep, almost meaty flavour. This miso sauce, with its rich taste, can be used instead of high-fat gravies with poultry or game, and it is also an excellent accompaniment to rice, noodles, millet or bulgar wheat.

SERVES 2

1 tablespoon cold-pressed olive oil
1 onion, peeled and chopped
½ bunch watercress
1 carrot, grated
2 level tablespoons wholewheat plain flour
600 ml (1 pint) water
1 tablespoon miso, diluted with 2 tablespoons of water
2 spring onions, trimmed and chopped
2 tablespoons chopped fresh parsley

Heat the oil and sauté the onion for 2 minutes. Add the watercress, then the carrot and sauté for another 5 minutes. Sprinkle with the flour and cook for 5 minutes, stirring constantly. Gradually add the water and bring to the boil, stirring continuously. Add the diluted miso and simmer for another 5 minutes. Before serving stir in the spring onions and parsley.

SIMPLE MISO SAUCE

Faster to prepare than the previous version, this is delicious with wholegrains, tofu and Quorn. I use it with brown rice and cooked strips of nori seaweed (see page 136).

SERVES 2

1 heaped tablespoon miso
4 tablespoons tahini
250 ml (8 fl oz) water
1 teaspoon grated orange peel (optional)
Few leaves of fresh basil (optional)

Mix the miso, tahini and water together thoroughly in a small pan. Cover and cook over a low heat for 15 minutes, stirring occasionally. Add the orange peel and basil, if using.

NO-COOK SWEET AND SOUR SAUCE

This is a quick version of this pungent sauce which works well as a marinade for tofu, white fish or chicken pieces.

SERVES 2

2 tablespoons live, low-fat yoghurt
1 tablespoon clear honey
1½ tablespoons cider vinegar

Blend all the ingredients together until smooth. If using as a marinade let the ingredients marinate for at least 2–3 hours before cooking.

SWEET AND SOUR SAUCE

Kuzu is available from health food shops. Produced from a Japanese root, it is easily digested and is a versatile alternative as a thickening agent.

SERVES 2–4

275 ml (9 fl oz) water, or stock or tomato juice
40 g (1½ oz) clear honey
135 ml (4½ fl oz) cider vinegar
2 tablespoons cornflour, or kuzu or arrowroot, blended
    with a little cold water
1 dessertspoon tamari sauce
Freshly ground black pepper or a dash of Tabasco sauce

Optional extra seasonings
Garlic, fresh root ginger, dark sesame oil or
    Worcestershire sauce to taste

Heat the water, stock or tomato juice with the honey and vinegar. When boiling, add the blended cornflour, kuzu or arrowroot. Add the tamari sauce, and freshly ground black pepper or Tabasco sauce to taste. Add one or more of the extra seasonings, if using.

HUMUS SAUCE

MAKES 400 ML (14 FL OZ)

225 g (8 oz) cooked chick peas (see page 74)
2 cloves garlic, peeled and crushed
1 tablespoon tahini
3–4 leaves fresh basil
250 ml (8 fl oz) cold water

In a food processor, purée the chick peas with the garlic, tahini and basil to obtain a smooth paste. Alternatively, mash the ingredients together in a large bowl using a potato masher. Thin the paste to the consistency of a sauce by adding enough cold water.

RAW APPLE SAUCE

A versatile recipe that is truly delicious with Buckwheat pancakes (page 166).

SERVES 2–4

4 eating apples, cored and chopped (preferably unpeeled)
Juice of ½ lemon
A little grated nutmeg
A pinch of cinnamon
50–100 ml (2–4 fl oz) apple juice

Blend the apples with the lemon juice and spices in a food processor. Add sufficient apple juice to achieve the desired consistency. The sauce may be warmed through gently in a small saucepan if preferred, but do not let it boil.

Kiddies' Corner

Children are notoriously hard to please, but these recipes seem to satisfy the fussiest eaters.

FISH CAKES

This recipe works well with cod, coley and hoki (an inexpensive New Zealand fish available at most supermarkets), or try it with salmon for the grown-ups!

MAKES 8 FISH CAKES

550 g (1¼ lb) potatoes, scrubbed
4 tablespoons cold-pressed olive oil
Freshly ground black pepper
1 large onion, peeled and finely chopped
450 g (1 lb) fresh (or frozen and defrosted) cod, coley or hoki
    fillets
1 tablespoon fresh thyme, chopped
Juice of ½ lemon
1 free-range egg, size 3, lightly beaten
4–6 tablespoons sesame seeds for coating

Boil the potatoes until cooked, drain and mash them with 1 tablespoon of olive oil and freshly ground black pepper to season. Heat another tablespoonful of olive oil and fry the onion and fish until the fish is white and the onion is transparent. Mix the fish and onion with the mashed potato and add the thyme, lemon juice and egg, stirring well.

Mould the mixture into 8 round, flat fish cakes. Coat with the sesame seeds. Heat the remaining olive oil and fry the fish cakes for a few minutes on each side until golden brown.

BAKED BEANS

SERVES 4–6

1 tablespoon olive oil for frying
1 onion, peeled and finely chopped
100 g (4 oz) bacon, rinded and chopped (optional)
450 g (1 lb) fresh tomatoes, skinned, deseeded and chopped
or 400 g (1 × 14 oz) tin chopped tomatoes
2 teaspoons tomato purée
2 teaspoons chopped fresh basil
250 g (9 oz) dried haricot beans, soaked in water overnight,
    drained and cooked in water for 50–60 minutes
or 400 g (2 × 14 oz) tins of haricot beans

Heat the olive oil and fry the onion and bacon (if using) until the
onion is transparent. Add the tomatoes and cook gently until they
become a pulp. Stir in the tomato purée and the basil. Drain and
add the beans and cook for several minutes until heated through.

MILLET MASH

SERVES 3–4

1 teaspoon sesame oil or cold-pressed olive oil
1 medium onion, peeled and diced
1 tablespoon tamari sauce
175–225 g (6–8 oz) cauliflower or broccoli, cut into florets
200 g (7 oz) millet
600 ml (1 pint) water
1 tomato, chopped
1 sprig fresh parsley

Heat the oil and gently fry the onion until transparent. Stir in the
tamari sauce and add the cauliflower or broccoli, millet and water.
Bring to the boil briefly then cover and simmer until soft. Mash
until smooth. Serve with chopped tomatoes and fresh parsley.

BEAN AND FLOUR PATTIES

The gram flour used in this recipe comes from ground chick peas and gives the patties a distinctive flavour and golden colour.

MAKES APPROX. 14 PATTIES

100 g (4 oz) gram flour
About 300 ml (½ pint) skimmed, semi-skimmed or soya milk
1 tablespoon cold-pressed olive oil for frying
175 g (6 oz) cooked aduki beans
1 teaspoon each chopped fresh oregano, thyme and marjoram

Sieve the flour into a basin and stir in the milk, to make a light batter. Heat the oil in a frying pan and add spoonfuls of the batter. Sprinkle 2 teaspoons aduki beans on each pattie before turning to fry on the other side. Remove from the pan and keep the patties warm whilst you cook the remaining batter.

NO-COOK RISSOLES

Serve these rissoles with Vitamin salad (see page 177) or a green salad tossed with Yoghurt and chive dressing (see page 181).

MAKES 8 SMALL RISSOLES

175 g (6 oz) mixed nuts (e.g. hazelnuts and almonds), ground
100 g (4 oz) wholewheat breadcrumbs
1 dessertspoon finely chopped onion
1 tablespoon chopped parsley
1 teaspoon low-salt yeast extract blended with 1 tablespoon
    water
1 dessertspoon poppy or sesame seeds

Reserve about one-quarter of the nuts and breadcrumbs for coating, and mix all the remaining ingredients together. Form into small rissoles. Mix together the reserved nuts and bread-crumbs and use to coat the rissoles.

Perfect Puddings

You don't have to go without dessert to eat yourself beautiful! Many wholegrains combine well with naturally sweet fruits to make puddings that don't need any additional sugar.

APPLE CRUMBLE

Use eating apples for their natural sweetness. Serve the crumble hot with Apple sauce (see page 207).

SERVES 4

450 g (1 lb) eating apples, unpeeled, cored and sliced
1 teaspoon grated lemon rind
50 g (2 oz) wholewheat, plain flour
75 g (3 oz) rolled oats
65 ml (2½ fl oz) sesame or cold-pressed olive oil

Pre-heat the oven to 160°C, 325°F (gas mark 3).

Place the apples in a lightly oiled, shallow baking dish and sprinkle with the lemon rind. Sift the flour into a basin and stir in the oats. Add the olive or sesame oil and mix with a round-bladed knife until crumbly. Sprinkle the crumb mixture over the apples.

Bake for 30 minutes, or until the apples are tender.

APPLE SAUCE

300 ml (½ pint) apple juice
3 teaspoons kuzu or arrowroot, blended with 1 tablespoon
    water

Heat the apple juice, stir in the kuzu or arrowroot and simmer for
a few minutes, stirring, until the sauce has thickened.

STRAWBERRY SORBET

This recipe can be easily adapted for use with other soft fruits,
such as raspberries.

SERVES 4

450 g (1 lb) fresh strawberries
2 teaspoons clear honey (optional)
Juice of 1 large orange

Blend the ingredients together in a food processor until smooth.
Pour into a bowl or container and place in the freezing
compartment of the fridge (or in the freezer) for one hour.

Remove and allow the mixture to thaw a little, if necessary,
then beat well with a metal spoon to break up any ice crystals and
return the sorbet to the freezer for at least 5 hours. Allow to
soften at room temperature for half an hour before serving.

SPICED BANANAS

This recipe works well with pears too. Another way to make this dish is to bake the fruit in a pre-heated oven 180°C, 350°F (gas mark 4) for 15 minutes to soften it, before pouring on the sauce and serving. Bake the bananas in their skins and they'll keep their colour better.

SERVES 4

4 large ripe bananas
50 g (2 oz) butter or soya margarine
1 tablespoon clear honey
2 teaspoons allspice

Peel and slice the bananas and place in four individual serving bowls. In a small saucepan quickly melt the butter or soya margarine, and stir in the honey and allspice. Pour over the bananas and serve immediately.

NICE RICE PUDDING

This wonderfully warming pudding gets most of its sweetness from the sweet brown rice. It is important to use pre-cooked rice.

SERVES 4

100 g (4 oz) cooked sweet brown rice
½ tablespoon clear honey or ½ tablespoon dried fruit,
    such as sultanas, chopped apricots or dates
600 ml (1 pint) soya milk
Pinch of freshly grated nutmeg

Pre-heat the oven to 150°C, 300°F (gas mark 2).
    Place the pre-cooked rice in a lightly oiled ovenproof dish. Stir the honey or the dried fruit into the milk and pour over the rice. Sprinkle the fresh nutmeg on top. Bake for approximately two hours.

COURGETTE AND CARROT CAKE

This rich, dark cake tastes so delicious you won't believe it's so good for you! Less sweet than conventional recipes, it is enriched with vitamin E and iron. Butter is replaced with healthier mono-unsaturated oil which also makes the mixture fabulously moist. I add coarsely chopped walnut pieces for extra crunch, but if baking for small children these should be finely ground to avoid the risk of choking. I find that dipping the spoon into hot water before spooning out the molasses and honey enables these sticky sweeteners to slide off the spoon more easily.

MAKES TWO 18 CM (7 INCH) CAKES

2 free-range eggs, size 3
2 tablespoons crude blackstrap molasses
2 tablespoons clear honey
150 ml (¼ pint) plus 1 tablespoon walnut, hazelnut
    or olive oil
175 g (6 oz) buckwheat flour
1 teaspoon bicarbonate of soda
50 g (2 oz) natural wheatgerm
50 g (2 oz) chopped walnuts
100 g (4 oz) carrots, scrubbed and grated
100 g (4 oz) courgettes, washed and grated
4 tablespoons orange juice

Pre-heat the oven to 180°C, 350°F (gas mark 4).
    Lightly oil two Victoria sandwich tins with the 1 tablespoon of oil. In a large mixing bowl, beat the eggs together before adding the molasses and honey. Stir vigorously before pouring in 150 ml (¼ pint) oil. Fold in the buckwheat flour, bicarbonate of soda and wheatgerm, followed by the remaining ingredients. Pour into the baking tins and bake for 35–40 minutes, or until a metal skewer comes out clean. Allow to cool before turning out and slicing into wedges. Store in a tightly sealed container in a cool place.

Useful Addresses

Food Additives is the best booklet on food additives and their potential health risks. Supported by the BBC's *Good Food* magazine, this is an essential shopping guide and costs £2 from:
The Food Commission
88 Old Street
London EC1V 9AR
071 253 9513

Action & Information on Sugars
28 St Paul Street
London N1
Written enquiries only

British Herbal Medicine Association
Field House
Lye Hole Lane
Redhill
Avon BS18 7TB
0934 862994
New members welcome. Can advise of your nearest qualified herbal practitioner or stockist of herbal remedies.

British Register of Naturopathy
328 Harrogate Road
Moortown
Leeds LS17 6PE
Send an SAE for details of your nearest registered naturopath or details of naturopathy training.

Coeliac Society
PO Box 220
High Wycombe
Buckinghamshire HP11 2HY
Publish a regularly up-dated list of gluten-free manufactured products. Please send an SAE for more information. Written enquiries only.

Community Health Foundation
188 Old Street
London EC1V 9FR
071 251 4076
Macrobiotic and vegetarian cookery classes (full-time, evenings and weekends). Courses on shiatsu massage, T'ai Chi, yoga and many more healing arts. Also the home of Britain's largest macrobiotic restaurant.

The Food Commission
88 Old Street
London EC1V 9AR
071 253 9513
This watchdog organisation provides independently researched information on foods and publishes The Food Magazine *quarterly.*

Foresight
The Old Vicarage
Church Lane
Witley
Godalming
Surrey GU8 5PN
0428 684500
The association for the promotion of pre-conceptual care. Funds research into infertility and birth defects resulting from poor nutrition and offers practical advice for would-be parents.

General Council and Register of Osteopaths
56 London Street
Reading
Berkshire RG1 4SQ
0734 576585
Send an SAE for details of your nearest registered osteopath or details of osteopathy training.

Henry Doubleday Research Association
Bocking
Braintree
Essex CV8 3LG
0203 303517
Largest organisation of organic gardeners in the world and new members are welcome. Specialises in research into comfrey. Products and gardening books available by mail order.

The Society of Herbalists
77 Great Peter Street
London SW1P 2E2
Written enquiries only.

National Food Alliance
102 Gloucester Place
London W1H 3DA
071 935 2889
An association of voluntary, professional, health, consumer and other organisations that aims to develop food and agriculture policies to the benefit of public health.

Quitline
071 487 3000
The smoker's helpline for friendly advice and helpful tips if you are planning to give up smoking or need additional encouragement while quitting. Quitline can also put you in touch with self-help groups and offer an advice service for GPs planning stop-smoking sessions. Funded by the Health Education Authority. 9.30–5.30 Monday to Friday.

SAFE (Sustainable Agriculture, Food and Environment)
21 Tower Street
London WC2H 9NS
071 240 1811
The SAFE alliance represents more than 20 organisations and has European contacts. Campaign packs are available from the above address.

The Soil Association
86 Colston Street
Bristol BS1 5BB
0272 290661
Their symbol is a consumer guarantee that food is high quality and genuinely organically grown. The Soil Association welcomes new members and can also advise on stockists of organically grown produce.

The Vegetarian Society
Parkdale
Dunham Road
Altrincham
Cheshire WA14 4QG
061 928 0793

World Cancer Research Fund
Freepost CV1037
Stratford-upon-Avon CV37 0BR
This charity studies the effects of diet on cancer. A booklet entitled ABC Guide To Reducing Your Cancer Risk is available free from the above address. Written enquiries only.

Suppliers

Clearspring
Extensive mail order selection of foods (including macrobiotic ingredients), cookware and books. For a price list contact
Clearspring Mail Order
5–10 Eastman Road
London W3 7YG
081 746 2261

Clearspring Natural Grocer
196 Old Street
London EC1V 9BP
Britain's largest macrobiotic grocer and stockist of a wide range of seaweeds, rices, wholegrains and organic foods. Also books and cookware. Well worth a visit – but allow plenty of time to browse. Many of the foods may be tasted in the macrobiotic restaurant next door at 188 Old Street.

Organic Food Market
Spitalfields, gates 8–9
Commercial Street
London E1
071 286 9204
Modelled on the popular French Marché Biologique, this market opens on Sundays from 9 am to 3 pm and has many stalls selling organic produce of every description.

Natural Foods
Unit 14
The Sidings
Hainault Road
London E11 1HD
081 539 1034 (for an extensive price list)
Britain's largest home-delivery service for high quality organic produce including free-range and organic meat, fish and seafood from non-polluted sources, organic herbs, wines and environmentally friendly household supplies. Deliveries anywhere within greater London, Essex and Hertfordshire. Will also Red Star or post further afield. Helpful, friendly service.

The Watermill
Mail order suppliers of organic, stoneground flours by post. Will also post organic cereal products, wholegrains, dried fruits, nuts, seeds and herb teas. For a catalogue contact The Watermill, Little Salkeld, Penrith, Cumbria CA10 1NN.
0768 881523.

Wholefood
071 935 3924 (for Mail order details)
24 Paddington Street
London W1M 4DR
The first shop to supply a wide range of organic produce, Wholefood also stocks an extensive range of food and supplements. Also an extensive selection of books and journals on health, nutrition, organic farming and gardening. Organic meat also available from 31 Paddington Street.

Notes on the Text

1 Studies at the Technion-Israel Institute of Technology, Haifa and at the Department of Biochemistry and Medicine, Bone and Connective Tissue Research Laboratory, University of Southern California have found that substances in avocados are able to block the enzyme *lysyl oxidase* which inhibits the formation of soluble collagen as we age.

2 Studies include a trial involving lung cancer patients at The Johns Hopkins University School of Hygiene and Public Health in 1986; colon, lung and stomach cancer patients involved in the Japan-Hawaii Cancer Study, Hawaii in 1985 and breast cancer patients at The Cancer Epidemiology and Clinical Trials Unit, Radcliffe Infirmary, Oxford in 1984. In 1991, more general studies reported in the *American Journal of Epidemiology* also confirmed that cancer patients had low beta carotene levels in their blood.

3 Professor Micheline Matthews-Roth of Harvard Medical School has spent over twenty years studying the effects of beta carotene on the skin. As a result of her research, the antioxidant is now approved by the United States Food and Drug Administration (FDA) for the specific treatment of light-sensitive skin disorders. Professor Matthews-Roth's research has also confirmed that beta carotene plays a significant part in preventing sunburn whilst we are exposed to the sun.

4 One example of the importance of vitamin E was highlighted by a study into breast cancer carried out at the Radcliffe Infirmary, Oxford in 1984 which concludes 'the risk of breast cancer in women with vitamin E levels in the lowest quintile was about five times higher than the risk for women with levels in the highest quintile'. In other words, a low quota of vitamin E in our food is a considerable health risk.

5 A paper published by The Food Commission in 1991 reports that women on low incomes are most at risk from iron deficiency and that while a diet containing 10 mg iron per 1000 kcals is advised, many women are actually eating nearer 6 mg iron per 1000 kcals.

6 Amongst the most recent clinical trials to confirm the effects of fish oils on the skin was a double-blind clinical trial by Dr Vincent A. Ziboh at the Department of Dermatology, University of California in 1991. After a period of eight weeks, those suffering from skin disorders who were taking fish oil capsules reported less itching, redness and inflammation compared to those taking dummy capsules. Subsequent trials carried out at the Department of Dermatology, Queen's Medical Centre, Nottingham, confirm that fish oils can improve the condition and appearance of with severe disorders such as psoriasis.

7 Dr James E. Rasmussen is based at the Department of Dermatology, State University of New York at Buffalo School of Medicine, New York.

7a According to studies by Drs Lewellyn and MacDonald, recorded in the *Journal of Investigative Dermatology* (1966) and the *British Journal of Dermatology* (1967) respectively.

8 A study in the medical journal *The Lancet* in 1988 reported that migraine sufferers are particularly susceptible to migraine attacks after drinking wine. Nine out of the eleven sufferers tested found that wine triggered migraine while vodka mixed to the same alcoholic strength did not.

9 A double-blind study by Dr Neil Ward published in the *Journal of Nutritional Medicine* in 1990 shows that when just 200 ml (⅓ pint) of a tartrazine-coloured, orange drink was given to hyperactive children, their behaviour and emotional responses deteriorated rapidly. A staggering 30 per cent of these children also developed eczema or asthma within 30–40 minutes of drinking the squash.

Other titles available from the BBC:

The Well-Woman by Dr Margery Morgan

Assertiveness: The Right to be You by Calire Walmesly

Relax: Dealing with Stress by Murray Watts and Professor Cary L. Cooper

Sarah Brown's Healthy Pregnancy: A Vegetarian Approach

INDEX

INDEX

manganese, 26, 113
mange tout, 130
mango, 100
margarine, 43
marjoram, 158
marrows, 133
meat, 17–18, 43
melons, 100–1
methionine, 28
milk, 18, 23
millet, 65
  millet croquettes, 192
  millet mash, 204
minerals, 22–4, 113
mint, 158
miso sauce, 199–200
molasses, 47
monounsaturated fats, 31, 142, 146
mucus, 23–4
muesli, Bircher, 168
mung beans, 74
mushrooms, 127
  asparagus and mushroom risotto, 195
  mushroom pâté, 173
mustard, 119
  creamy mustard sauce, 197

naturopaths, 23
nightshade family, 120–3
nitrates, 113
nori, 136–7
nutmeg, 161–2
nuts, 14, 78–80
  no-cook rissoles, 205

oats, 14, 66
oils, 17
  herb oils, 154–5
  plant oils, 139–51
olive oil, 14, 139, 146, 147, 148–9
olives, tapenade, 191
onions, 130–1
  onion soup, 172
  tofu and onion flan, 186
oranges, 95–6
  orange and tamari dressing, 182
oregano, 158
organic vegetables, 112–13, 116–17

pancakes, buckwheat, 166
pantothenic acid, 20
papain, 29
papaya, 102
paprika, 162
parsley, 158
parsnips, 129
passion fruit, 102–3
pâté, mushroom, 173
patna rice, 70
paw paw, 102
peaches, 103–4
peanuts, 80
pearl barley, 62
pears, 104
peas, 129–30
  dried peas, 74
pectin, 14, 89
peppercorns, 162
peppers, 122–3
peptic ulcers, 14
pesticides, 39, 60, 112–13, 114–16
phenylalanine, 29
phosphorus, 22–3
pineapples, 105
plant oils, 139–51
plums, 105
polenta, 65
polyunsaturated fats, 31, 142, 146
poppy seeds, 162
pork: home-made herb sausages, 183
pot barley, 62
potassium, 24, 41
potatoes, 17, 121–2
prawn kebabs with herb dressing, 196
prostaglandins, 143–4, 145
protein, 113
prunes, 105–6
pudding rice, 70
puddings, 206–9
pulses, 72–4
pumpkin seeds, 75–6

quinoa, 66–7

radishes, 127
rapeseed oil, 149
raspberries, 107
raw food, 117–18

222

INDEX